SEXUAL ANXIETY
A Study of Male Impotence

SEXUAL ANXIETY
A Study of Male Impotence

ERIC CARLTON

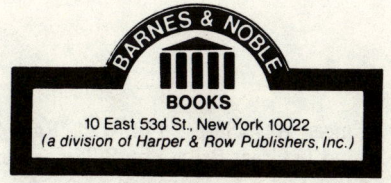

© Eric Carlton 1980

All rights reserved. No part of this publication may be reproduced, stored in a retrieval system, or transmitted in any form or by any means, electronic, mechanical, photocopying, recording or otherwise without the prior written permission of the copyright holder.

First published in 1980 by Martin Robertson & Co. Ltd., 108 Cowley Road, Oxford OX4 1JF.

Published in the U.S.A. 1980 by Harper & Row Publishers, Inc., Barnes & Noble Import Division.

ISBN 0-06-490960-3
LC 79-56651

RC
560
.I45
C37
1980

Typeset by Pioneer Associates, Flimwell, East Sussex.
Printed and bound in Great Britain by Billing & Sons Ltd., Guildford, London, Oxford, Worcester.

Contents

Preface vii

Introduction 1

1. Definitions of Impotence 9
2. The Concept of Sexual Normality 27
3. The Incidence of Impotence I:
   Some Comparative and Historical Perspectives 51
4. The Incidence of Impotence II:
   The Current Situation 65
5. Case Histories 77
6. Theories of Male Sexual Dysfunction 101
7. Sex Therapies 127
8. Some Conclusions 159
   Notes 179
   Bibliography 187
   Index 195

Preface

The 'real' situation concerning male impotence is quite unknown. There are a few statistics, but these are little more than intelligent guesses. For example, one particular pilot study (Nichols, 1961) showed that 52% of the married men interviewed had unsatisfactory sexual relationships, but the sample was small, and the causes remained indefinite. Subjective impressions had led some earlier investigators to the conclusion that most men experience some kind of dysfunction sometime in their lives, but, again, there is no certainty on the issue (e.g. Jones, 1918). And whether impotence is primarily organic or psychogenic in origin is also still in dispute (Cooper *et al.*, 1970). All one can do is to make reasonable inferences from the limited research findings which are available.

Yet a further problem is the nature of the sources themselves. Obviously these authorities cannot all carry equal weight. Some are highly reputable, usually specialists operating in the field of sex therapy. Others are rather more uncertain, and doubts remain as to the methods of investigation and the processing of the statistics.

This particular study has been conducted at four levels:

(1) The analysis of specialist literature, much of which is not yet known to, or even available to the layman.
(2) Discussions with specialists — particularly therapists — working in the subject area.

(3) A content analysis of popular press and periodical material, particularly women's magazines and explicit 'fringe' literature. Much of this material may seem 'light' and unsophisticated, but it does reflect everyday concerns, and should not be ignored.
(4) Case studies that were personally conducted, and which have never been reported in any other books or journals.

This rather catholic approach to the problem may only partly meet the rigorous experimental standards demanded by some practitioners, but it does give a *composite* view which should illuminate the main issues for the general reader.

This study began with the suicide of a friend, and it is to his memory that this book is dedicated.

Introduction

In a recent discussion of sexual problems at a symposium held in San Francisco, the Director of the National Sex Forum, the Reverend Edward McIlvenna, maintained that male impotence is the 'primary sex problem of modern society'. He even went further and hypothesized that sex crime and violence are expressions of a 'warped mentality' which itself derives from 'the lack of release to which all are entitled'.

This sentiment reflects a particular view of the sex instinct to which not everyone would subscribe. But it also highlights the subject of impotence, which, as a problem, is yet to be clearly defined. Current evaluations have concentrated on biochemical and psychological interpretations for both explanatory and therapeutic purposes. A broader approach — perhaps more sociologically oriented — may be required to extend, and perhaps even to correct, our understanding of the condition. This particular discussion of impotence, however, does not pretend to be a sociological analysis, but it will be informed by a sociological perspective. In this way, it is hoped to complement the popular psychosexual approach and to refine some of the traditional notions of sexuality.

Before the modern publication of such exotica as *The Perfumed Garden* and the *Karma Sutra*, the first serious attempts to plot patterns of sexual behaviour were made towards the end of the nineteenth century with the pioneer works of Krafft-Ebing and the unlikely Havelock-Ellis.

The most obvious people to grapple with the problems of sexual pathology were the medical experts, but they were soon joined by the confident devotees of the newly emergent science of psychology.

Today, sex has become the subject of careful scrutiny by academics and health professions. It has always been open to the de-sanctifying influences of ribald humour, but now its ecstasies are being clinically neutralized by all manner of psycho-medical investigations. Some might argue that sex should not be the object of these doubtful theoretical concerns which are considered to be both illconceived and unrewarding. Others might go further and contend that such appraisals involve mechanistic evaluations which can actually inhibit normal sex performance. After all, nothing destroys an experience more quickly than subjecting it to analytical study; its nuances die in the very act of dissection.

Until relatively recently sex had been one of those less contentious areas where tradition enjoyed a large measure of general agreement. Our very existence suggests that its applications were reasonably effective. True, it had its quota of old wives' tales and quasi-religious superstitions; but, if anything, these added to its attractions. For most of history, the enjoyment of sex had escaped the de-mystifying implications of the theorists, and its practitioners remained untouched by the unromantic ministrations of the professional therapists. But the sublimities that were once applauded by bards and poets are now yielding to analysis. The private experience has become titillatingly public. Open rehearsals can now be traced from the academic to the exhibitionistic, from 'doctors" books to the 'experience' magazines. From there it is but a short step to the merely platitudinous — to the ultimate indignities of the 'problem page'.

But is all this really necessary? Don't we all know about sex? Naturally, commonsense appreciations of sex are not to be ignored, but that does not mean that they cannot be questioned. Here we are faced with the problem of conflicting rationalities. What makes sexual sense to one person does not always make sense to another. And this is even more true of different cultures. Commonsense tends to vary with the context in which it is expressed. What, for example, can Western rationality make of the economics of Indian temple prostitution or the Phoenician custom whereby occasional prostitution becomes a ritual act — almost like a Muslim going to Mecca? Or how is sophisticated man going to interpret such bizarre sexual behaviour as clitorodectomy (female circumcision) found traditionally in some African tribes, and the virility contests that have been reported among some Sudanese peoples? Both practices are strange by Western standards, but both may well be indirectly related to potency fears. Modern society may consider these alien and even abhorrent, but then it tends to substitute its own particular brands of sexual diversion, and these are not rationalized in terms of lofty ritual imperatives but in the earthier language of self-expression and liberation.

So how reliable *are* commonsense explanations? Is the public really in need of sexual instruction, and how necessary are the 'experts' to our understanding of what seem to be essentially 'natural' issues? Obviously, commonsense views must be given their due, but this does not imply that they are inherently superior to those of the professional. On the other hand, the professional must not discount the given elements that are found in naturalistic perceptions of a situation. For though so-called natural explanations imply a common knowledge of how people react in given situations, they cannot give us either a clearly delineated sample of people in those situations, or coherent explanations as to why such situations occur. So in the case of sexual impotence, traditional knowledge may not, of itself, be capable of identifying the causes or designing the therapies. This does not mean that it should be disparaged as fit only for the simpleminded. Sometimes, the theory that the professional substitutes for the everyday explanation is no more than a banal generalization which adds little to our real understanding of the situation. There is always too the professional penchant for seeing hidden reasons for things that are cryptically concealed from the uninitiated. Only the theoretically sophisticated discern the true meanings: people vote Conservative because they were denied the left breast as children, or strike — not for more money or shorter working hours — but because they are making a belated protest against parental authority.

It follows, therefore, that the accumulated lore of the past often has some basis in experience, and is therefore not always to be despised. But it must be looked at critically, and — where possible — it must be refined by more rigorous forms of analysis.

In social investigation it may not be possible to say anything particularly original. In fact, there is a sense in social research in which nothing is original and everything is original. Human activity is forever concerned with the singular and the unique. But, at the same time, human behaviour is patterned behaviour which is amenable to certain generalized forms of analysis. Social scientists do uncover 'new' facts which are sometimes statable in numerical terms; but by and large they are more concerned to offer alternative interpretations of perennial problems. The data themselves do not constitute social knowledge, and the collection of data is not to be equated with social science. So this discussion will be concerned not only with facts but also with *meanings*. It is a 'fact' that we all inherit certain physical forms and a variety of biological limitations, but we are also legatees of a socially constructed world which becomes a major determinant of our experience. This is a world of received sexual norms and values, and we will begin to understand impotence only when we come to appreciate the meanings with which sex is endowed in our own and in other societies.

In general, therefore, this study of impotence necessarily involves some consideration of broader issues associated with patterns of sexual behaviour. These need to be re-evaluated for a number of reasons. There still exists, for instance, the necessity of trying to balance certain persuasive contending views of sex. The emphasis of biological determinism, supported by the apparent validations of behavioural psychology, tends to give rise to the idea of sex as an inner eruptive force which must be canalized and regulated by the individual and society. On the other hand, there is the notion — associated with more radical sexual ideologies — that sex is a universal panacea whose uninhibited expression inevitably leads to ultimate social and personal fulfillment. This increasingly popular view of sex as the source of final liberation was once regarded as just one more idiosyncracy of the protest spectrum. Now it finds more socially acceptable advocates who insist that sexual expression is controlled by traditional institutions in the mistaken interests of social order.

A study of impotence, therefore, not only is interesting in itself, but it also highlights certain features of the changing attitudes on sexual matters. It must be concerned with modes of cultural transmission; learning processes are important, although they obviously cannot be divorced from the limitations of physical inheritance. So, unfashionable as it is in social science, some deference to biological functionalism must be accepted. After all, only in a highly qualified sense can impotence be regarded as subjectively problematic. Some consideration too will be given to the matter of sex therapy. This requires critical appraisal, as there may be some relationship between the development of sexological theory and counselling agencies and the actual emergence of practical difficulties. In addition, the examination of the 'grey areas' of sexual practice tends to throw into relief the disparities between the ideal and the actual, and, therefore, has possible implications for either the easing or tightening of moral strictures and even legal constraints on particular categories of sexual behaviour.

Even though, sociologically speaking, sexual activity in modern society is primarily recreational, from a biological point of view it is still primarily procreational. This study takes the biological frameworks as given; it adopts the perspective of the sympathetic reactionary. Nevertheless, it does stress the crucial role of 'understanding' in relation to sexual problems. Its orientation, then, is generally conservative, and it avoids the overcharted areas of sexual politics, except as the arguments of liberation movements inevitably impinge upon theories of impotence. Homosexuality too tends to be disregarded, but this is largely because it appears to be greatly underrepresented in the available data, and because the general points which are made about impotence apply equally to homosexuals and heterosexuals alike.

The book is really addressed to that rather shadowy figure, the intelligent layman, although it is hoped that it will also be interesting and provocative enough to appeal to professionals such as social workers, counsellors, etc. It assumes a critical stance, and is often prepared to make certain value judgements. Because there are serious limits to which a study of sexual dysfunction can be treated as just another social survey, a case study approach has been adopted where necessary. In general, however, it is an examination of a complex psycho-sexual phenomenon looked at from a number of different points of view. There is no *one* overriding perspective, no one answer, no particular 'case' to be made. It is a search for possibilities rather than an attempt to advance any main argument or establish any particular theory. To approach it as a thesis would mean artificially reducing the actual complexities to rule, and this would ignore the confusing nature of the reality.

1. Definitions of Impotence

The term 'impotence' is sometimes regarded as both vague and objectionable (Kaplan, 1974, p.256). Vague because, almost incredibly, impotence eludes any really satisfactory definition, and objectionable because it has pejorative connotations. The former can be sharpened by some form of definitional analysis — that is to say, by a consideration of the *circumstances* in which a man may be thought of as impotent. But presumably the latter can be changed only by a gradual process of re-education.

Largely because of casual usage, the term 'impotence' lacks precision. It is still used to cover a number of different conditions which are thought to be related: ejaculatory impotence, premature ejaculation and — most commonly — erectile impotence (Brecher, 1972, pp.152-3).

(1) Ejaculatory impotence is the condition where a male is unable to ejaculate during intercourse, and sometimes achieves his orgasm afterwards by masturbation. This appears to be a relatively rare condition; Kinsey found only six reported cases in 4108 respondents (Kinsey *et al.,* 1948).

(2) Premature ejaculation usually indicates the condition where the male ejaculates either before or immediately after intromission. In considering the 'normality' or otherwise of this situation, it is probably worth noting Kinsey's observation (Kinsey *et al.,* 1948) that, for

perhaps as many as three-quarters of all males, 'orgasm is reached within two minutes after the initiation of the sexual relation, and for a not inconsiderable number ... the climax may be reached within less than a minute or even within ten or twenty seconds after coital entrance'. Arguably, Kinsey refused to recognize that premature ejaculation was really a *problem* for the male, although he conceded that it probably presented difficulties for his partner. Writing very much as a zoologist, he tended to take the view that rapid ejaculation is typical of male mammals generally, and that this rapidity and intensity of response — found particularly among higher primates — was something that might be 'labelled ... superior' (Kinsey *et al.,* 1948).

(3) Erectile impotence denotes either the inability to achieve an erection or the inability to maintain it until orgasm. This is much less rare than ejaculatory impotence,[1] and can obviously be operationally related to premature ejaculation, which may occur simultaneously with the loss of erection.

These various conditions sometimes yield to similar therapies, but each may be occasioned by quite different factors. To substitute — as some do (Masters and Johnson, 1966) — the more general expression 'male sexual inadequacy' to encompass all these symptoms is even less clinically neutral. It tends to pre-judge the issue as to exactly what is — or can be — meant by sexual adequacy and inadequacy. Similar reservations apply to other commonly used terms such as 'sexual malfunction' or 'sexual dysfunction', which, though virtually unavoidable, also assume what normality of function really is. This will be a crucial feature of the following discussion. What precisely do we mean by normality, and how can this be assessed?

It should be reiterated that impotence, by definition, is exclusively a male problem. That is to say, it should not be seen as the male counterpart of female frigidity. Obviously, they have affinities, but they should not — for very fundamental reasons — be regarded as complementary aspects of the same phenomenon. Perhaps the condition commonly termed 'frigidity' deserves some consideration in this context if only to point up its dissimilarities with male impotence.

Frigidity, which relates to the female, is yet another confusing term which covers a variety of phenomena. At the most general level, it refers to the apparent inability of a woman to respond to sexual stimulation. More specifically, it may be used to denote the failure of a woman to experience orgasm. Between these extremes are a host of intermediate positions: the woman who finds pleasure in sexual activity but who is inorgasmic; the woman who can obtain intense satisfaction from manual or mechanical stimulation, but who finds actual intercourse painful, difficult or even objectionable; and other assorted variants. Some women, possibly for either physiogenic or psychogenic reasons, may be put in a 'primary frigidity' category if they have never experienced sexual arousal, while others may be classified under the heading of 'secondary frigidity' if they once enjoyed such experiences but no longer do so.

Defined as loosely as this, the term 'frigidity' can include almost every shade of female sexual non-experience. If on the other hand strict physiological criteria are applied, and attempts are made to assess degrees of sexual excitation in terms of genital vasocongestion, (the engorgement of the blood vessels) or myotonia (muscle tension), problems still remain. A woman may experience orgasm by manual stimulation or mechanically by vibrator without the swelling of the labia and the vaginal tissues, or the lubrication of the vagina, all of which are normally associated with sexual excitation (Kaplan, 1974, p.362). And the situation is made even more problematic by the complex nature of the female orgasm itself. Research indicates that it consists of four main phases; excitement, plateau, orgasm and resolution.[2] In the orgasmic phase proper, the actual intensity of experience can vary considerably. Under laboratory conditions, it has been shown that a mild orgasm may be accompanied by only three to five vaginal contractions while in an intense orgasm this might be doubled or even trebled (Masters and Johnson, 1966). The orgasmic experience obviously varies from person to person, and even with the *same* person in differing circumstances. Indeed, in one extreme case, again recorded under laboratory conditions, Masters and Johnson mention a woman's orgasm which extended to twenty-five contractions lasting some forty-three seconds.

Given, therefore, the range and variability of the female orgasmic experience, it follows that the whole conception of frigidity as a condition is characterized by uncertainty and imprecision. In actual experiential — as opposed to experimental — situations, it can be extremely difficult both to assess and to classify the female response. Female excitation and female orgasm *in experiential conditions* are not subject to verification. The male partner can only know what she *appears* to feel or what she *says* she experiences. She may — perhaps for the very best motives — decide to deceive her partner. If so, there is no way in which he can possibly disprove or invalidate the 'experience'. Alternatively, she may not even understand or interpret her own experience correctly — whatever that may mean. But regardless of this, she can still give the *impression* of requited sexuality. There is no equivalent of ejaculatory impotence, premature ejaculation or erectile impotence for the female. The female response has a 'hidden-ness' that is ultimately inaccessible to the male. The female anatomy reflects this; the covert internality of the vagina involves a secret world of sexual possibilities. In the final analysis, the female sexual response is unknowable to the male.

This can never be so with the male. No male can will his own erection or his own ejaculation. He will either respond or not respond to the relevant stimuli. His response — or lack of it — can never be concealed. There are no possible ambiguities about male sexuality. It has an open irrefutability. Erectile potency or impotency is all too evident; there is a kind of sexual 'honesty' about the overt externality of the male genitalia that precludes even the possibility of deception. Either a man is excited or he is not, and his orgasm — which almost invariably culminates in ejaculation — is hardly a matter for interpretation.[3]

For the purposes of the present discussion, impotence — defined in medical terms[4] — may be taken to mean the conscious intention to attempt intercourse that fails for involuntary reasons. On this definition, therefore, it is very difficult to categorize as impotent the man who does not *try* to effect intercourse. But it includes failure to erect, failure to obtain a sufficiently hard erection to penetrate the vagina, loss of erection after penetration but before ejaculation, pre-penetration ejaculation and loss of erection, or ejaculation on intromission with consequent loss of erection (see Cauthery and Cole, 1971, p.188). This definitional framework does not include non-ejaculation, and it remains arguable whether it should also include so-called premature ejaculation, that is ejaculation soon after penetration, because — as we have seen from the Kinsey studies — the expression 'soon after penetration' is extremely relative and difficult to quantify. It can mean sooner than the subject intends, or sooner than his partner desires — or both. But it can be argued, as Kinsey tends to do (Kinsey *et al.*, 1948) that fairly rapid ejaculation is the 'natural' state of things, and that prolongation is simply a rather artificial sexual conceit of human society which has no really cogent biological justification. In the natural world, animals are most vulnerable during intercourse, and it can be speculated that rapid ejaculation developed as a form of survival mechanism. Certainly, as far as can be ascertained, impotence — as we have defined it — is unknown among animals (Cauthery and Cole, 1971, p. 189).

It should be noted that our definition of impotence does not include the absence, or apparent absence, of sexual *desire,* which may not be an incontravertible sign of impotence, but may merely denote the absence of the appropriate stimuli. Impotence, therefore, on our analysis involves the involuntary frustration of conscious sexual intentions that are usually — but not invariably — of a coital nature. Couched in these terms, it is a reasonable conjecture that most — if not all — men have experienced some kind of sexual dysfunction at some time in their lives (Cauthery and Cole, 1971, p. 188).

Any definition of impotence, therefore, must centre on the key problem of erectile dysfunction. Sustained and satisfactory erection is here taken as fundamental to all 'normal' male sexual activity. The matter of orgasmic and ejaculatory difficulty must, by this definition, take a secondary place. Of course, non-erection does not preclude the possibilities of sexual altruism; the male can always resort to manual or oral stimulation to excite his partner. But for his own potential orgasmic satisfaction, a sustained erection is the essential prerequisite.

Besides cataloguing the conditions to which the term 'impotence' is normally applied, there are other useful ways in which impotence can be classified. This is sometimes done in terms of convenient dichotomies. For example, Walker and Fletcher (1953) differentiate between organic and functional impotence. Organic impotence, which they regard as relatively rare except perhaps in elderly men, is impotence occasioned by some form of disease such as diabetes. The term 'functional impotence' they reserve for sexual dysfunction of a psychogenic nature. This is their primary concern, and they regard this as a very common condition, insisting that 'many reliable independent observations confirm [their] own conviction that no fewer than 90% of all men who seek medical and surgical treatment because their sexual powers have failed are suffering from [this] condition' (Walker and Fletcher, 1955, p. 160). Cauthery and Cole support this same general contention and insist that 95 per cent of all cases of impotence are of a psychological (i.e. functional) kind (Cauthery and Cole, 1971, p. 189).

A more fashionable distinction is that made by Masters and Johnson between primary and secondary impotence. They identify 'three major types of impotence ordinarily encountered in the human male' (Masters and Johnson, 1967, pp. 210-11):

(1) failed erection, i.e. where erection cannot be achieved;
(2) inadequate erection, i.e. erection that cannot be sustained;
(3) non-emissive erection, i.e. erection without ejaculation within the vagina.

These are re-classified as primary impotence, that is where erectile difficulties have always existed, and secondary impotence — which is much more common — where there has either been a change from erectile adequacy to erectile inadequacy or where erectile adequacy is punctuated by periods of inadequacy. The most unsatisfactory feature of this useful distinction is the somewhat arbitrary definition of inadequacy. Masters and Johnson have a rule-of-thumb method that suggests that for clinical purposes a man may be considered secondarily impotent if his attempts at intercourse fail in one out of four instances (Masters and Johnson, 1970, p. 157).

Of course, this kind of distinction cannot cover every

contingency. It says nothing about the situations in which secondary impotence is likely to occur, which can naturally vary from individual to individual. On the other hand, it has the merit of *not* assuming that there is some absolute scale against which all male performance can be evaluated. To 'calculate' secondary impotence on the basis of a 25 per cent failure rate means that a man's inadequacy is to be judged in terms of himself, and not in terms of some hypothesized overall standard. Obviously a man must maintain his erection long enough to penetrate the vagina and presumably reach a climax. Whether or not one should also include those who are potent in a variety of non-coital — possibly autoerotic — situations but who are unable to sustain an adequate erection for the actual coital act is a matter of some debate. Normally these are regarded as impotent,[5] but on the basis of our working definition it is arguable whether they should be. In the relevant literature there is the underlying assumption that judgements of male potency should be invariably based on *coital* performance with hypothetical women of average responsiveness. We all have vague ideas as to what such terms might mean in practice, but their vagueness certainly eludes any universally acceptable academic definitions.

As we have already noted, there is a fundamental similarity of sexual response in the male and the female, and these response patterns are generally independent of the type of stimulation or sexual activity that produces them (Masters and Johnson, 1966). The basic physiology of orgasm is the same, whether it is brought about by coitus, masturbation or whatever. The *type* of stimulation may affect the intensity of the responses to some extent, but they do not affect the fundamental changes that take place in the body.[6] However, there are a number of important dissimilarities which largely reflect anatomical differences.

First, it is perhaps necessary to reiterate the fact that

orgasm must not be confused with ejaculation. They are two separate processes. Orgasm can be experienced by both sexes and consists of a neuromuscular discharge of accumulated sexual tensions. Ejaculation, on the other hand, is experienced only by males following puberty when the prostate and accessory glands become functional. Females do not ejaculate; the fluid that lubricates the vagina is produced during arousal, and in no way corresponds to male semen.[7]

Second, although the orgasmic patterns of both sexes pass through the same general excitement, plateau, orgasm and resolution phases, the female cycle is subject to much more variability. The female orgasm may progress quickly — like that of the male — through each of the respective stages until the climax and resolution are obtained. Alternatively, sensation may mount rapidly to the plateau phase and be sustained for some time after which it is gradually dispersed in a more gentle 'rippled' climax. Or yet again, feelings may develop quickly and the final phases be experienced as an urgent orgasm or series of orgasms before the concluding resolution phase. Very generally speaking, the female response can be more ordered and controlled than that of the male, who can reach a point of no return at the onset of the orgasm stage when nothing can stop the ejaculation. After this, the male normally enters a 'refractory period', during which his erection subsides and in which he is therefore incapable of both intercourse and orgasm. When this period is over, he may then again be susceptible to sexual stimulation. (or perhaps the reverse is the case; when he becomes sensitive to stimulation the refractory period, by definition, can be said to be over. The research is not completely clear on this point.) The duration of the refractory period cannot be calculated with any real precision and varies from male to male and with the same male on different occasions. The age of the male, the frequency of sexual indulgence, the nature of the sexual stimuli, etc. — all these are factors that influence particular situations. But what can be said with some certainty is that, with few exceptions, the physiological ability of the male to respond to restimulation is lower than that of the female. She has no refractory periods, and therefore has the response potential of returning to yet further orgasmic experiences from any point of their resolution phase (Masters and Johnson, 1966, pp. 6-7). It is this capacity of women to experience multiple orgasms that can understandably prove rather daunting to even the super-potent male.

It had long been argued that women were capable of two main types of orgasm, centred either on the clitoris or on the vagina. This dual-orgasm hypothesis is particularly associated with Freud (1933), who argued that the clitoris is the site of immature sexual attention, and that after puberty the vagina should become the dominant orgasmic centre. If this transition does not occur, the woman concerned remains orgasmically undeveloped and possibly even frigid. Kinsey raised doubts about this hypothesis, and Masters and Johnson have confirmed in their researches that physiologically there is only *one* type of orgasm, and that the clitoris and the vagina respond identically. In practice, there may be tremendous variety in the subjective experience of orgasm. But this has an essentially psychological basis.[8] Regardless of the mode or site of stimulation, the actual physiological manifestations are much the same.

It would be a digression to explore here in any depth the clitoral-vaginal orgasm argument beloved of many Women's Liberationists.[9] They obviously appreciate the emancipatory possibilities inherent in clitoral supremacy, but they are not without their critics;[10] it may be based on false physiological premises. It has long been conceded that the vagina is not as sensitive as the clitoris. Kinsey found that in gynaecological examinations, 98 per cent of his subjects were able to perceive tactile stimulation of the clitoris, while only 14 per cent could detect being touched in the interior of the vagina (Kinsey *et al.,* 1953, pp. 574, 580). However, the Kinsey research team also encountered many women who claimed that deep vaginal penetration gave them a very special satisfaction which it is difficult to explain in *purely* psychological terms. The Freudian view that the centre of sensation is 'transferred' from the clitoris to the vagina is now considered *passé*. Similarly, the clitoral pre-eminence theory, which is still extremely popular, is undergoing some modification. Recent research evidence suggests that some form of theoretical rapprochement may be possible (e.g. Kaplan, 1974, pp. 27-32). The general consensus of opinion now tends to favour the view that the female orgasm is triggered by clitoral stimulation but expressed by vaginal contractions. The clitoris and the vagina, therefore, have complementary functions in the female orgasmic experience.[11]

A comparison of the male sexual response must involve some elementary discussion of the physiology of erection and ejaculation. First, it is important to note that erection and ejaculation are not invariably connected. It has been demonstrated clinically and experimentally that ejaculation may occur in the absence of erection. This can be achieved by 'artificial' stimulation of the appropriate cerebral centres;[12] in normal experience it can be seen in the phenomenon of nocturnal emissions (wet dreams), which may occur without any very marked erectile response. And certainly erection need not culminate in ejaculation, as the phenomenon of retarded ejaculation shows. This is more commonly an experience of the older man, who may 'enjoy love-play several times during the week, or even several times during one day, and be capable of achieving good erections each time. However, he will not be able nor feel the use to ejaculate as often' (Kaplan, 1974, pp. 20-1). This may, of course, free him from unnecessary concern, and even enhance his enjoyment of non-orgasmic sexuality. On the other hand, it is possible for males — again older males in particular — to experience a refractory period in which their erection subsides without having ejaculated, and they still may not be able to regain an erection for several hours.

Two underlying physiological mechanisms indicate the sex organs' response to simulation.[13] vasocongestion, the increased influx of blood to the tissues, and myotonia, increases in muscle tension which are particularly evident in orgasmic contractions.

ERECTION

Probably in all males erections occur from very early years. In infancy these may have nothing whatsoever to do with sexual stimulation. Of course, it can always be argued that, for example, the congestion of the penis that often takes place during sleep when the need to urinate is beginning to generate a dawning discomfort is really a form of subconscious sexuality. But such explanations have only a marginal, quasi-Freudian, plausibility. Kinsey *et al.* (1948, pp. 164-5) found that younger boys sometimes have erections in a wide variety of non-sexual yet emotionally charged situations which ranged from athletic activities to such things as coming home late and being chased by the police. It is not usually until the teens that boys' erectile responses develop more selective sexual patterns.

Although erections come in varying degrees of firmness, for convenience we should possibly define an erection as the enlargement and stiffening of the penis sufficient for sexual intercourse. There is no set time in which erections reach the necessary firmness. Individuals respond differently. Younger men are relatively quick, although slowing down with age may not be inevitable given that there are adequate stimuli. Erection has been termed the most delicate of the male sexual functions, and it is during this initial excitement phase of sexual activity — where there may be both a heightening and relaxation of emotional tension — that a man's erection is usually at its most vulnerable. It is at this time that the would-be lover probably requires experience and technique rather than sheer stamina.

Erection is essentially a vascular phenomenon that is triggered by a nervous reflex. Clinical evidence indicates that the rapid engorgement and disengorgement of the penis facilitated by the penile blood vessels is controlled by the autonomic nervous system centred in the spinal cord. These reflexes are involuntary in the sense that their response is automatic and does not require a 'decision' by the brain to effect the condition. Under normal circumstances[14] the brain is aware of these responses, which it can influence to a variable degree. The old adage that 'even a thought can lift a penis' is, of course, true. Fantasizing of an erotic nature can bring about an erection, but there is no certainty or invariability about this response, and certainly there is no way in which a man can 'order' his penis to respond in a particular way at a particular time. In fact, one disturbing feature that emerges from the treatment of erectile dysfunction is that the mind is as influential in inhibiting sexual responses as in exciting them. Indeed, it may well be that on occasions the body and the brain work against one another in this respect. The story is told of how Shaka, a despotic Zulu king in the early nineteenth century, tested the 'piety' of one of his regiments which had been deprived of sexual relations for some time. They were lined up naked while hundreds of scantily clad girls danced provocatively in front of them. Shaka — who may have been occasionally impotent himself — warned them that those who had erections would be executed. Many warriors began to erect despite their fears and were urged by some sympathetic girls to hit their own penises in order to detumesce rapidly, but — apparently — without much success (Becker, 1958, pp. 288-90).

We are reliably informed that 'Purely mental activity may thus trigger the mechanism of erection without physical stimulation, or it may inhibit erection despite physical stimulation' (Katchadourian and Lunde, 1972, p. 63). The problem here, however, is to know what pure mental activity can possibly be. The interactive process between 'pure' thought and bodily expression is something that is still very much under investigation. Mental images can induce erection, but an erection — or more likely a partial erection, which may have occurred for apparently non-sexual reasons — may itself act as the stimulus for a sequence of erotic thought which then reinforces the erection. It is well known that external sexual images, especially in films or magazines, may generate physical sexual activity; or, alternatively, physical activity — say, casual masturbation — may well stimulate sensual thoughts.

It is this problem of the relationship between the mind and the seemingly independent nervous system that is central to this entire discussion. We know that sexual response is not simply a mechanistic process. We know too that it involves neuro-physical operations of awesome complexity. But we are not sure just how, or to what extent, or even in what precise circumstances, conscious mental activity can affect sexual response. Paradoxically, the more autonomy these involuntary reflex actions possess, the less control men have over their own responses but the more chance there is of success for certain behavioural therapies. But we may not be completely at the mercy of pre-set neuro-physical forces, even if we cannot always help the way we react in sexual situations. Perhaps what we need to do is to explore the still somewhat uncharted areas of sexual socialization, and we may yet discover new dimensions of psycho-social importance.

Ejaculation

Although it is possible for the male to ejaculate without the 'full' orgasmic experience — as in 'wet dreams' — for all practical purposes ejaculation can be said to be synonymous with orgasm. Ejaculation, which again is a reflex action, takes place in two stages: emission, when the seminal fluid enters the urethra ready for discharge, and expulsion, when the fluid is discharged by vigorous contractions of the muscles at the base of the penis. The ejaculate itself, i.e. the seminal fluid, consists of spermatazoa (literally: 'seeds of life') and their medium of transmission, the fluid, consisting mainly of secretions from the prostate and the seminal vesicles, which makes up the bulk of the ejaculate. The volume of ejaculate varies, but seems usually to be about a teaspoonful (i.e. approximately 3 cubic centimetres), which will almost certainly diminish with close subsequent orgasms. The sperm count too will reduce with closely repeated ejaculations. The capacity to repeat the initial orgasm after only a short refractory period is usually construed as a sign of healthy sexuality — as indeed is the ability to delay ejaculation, which is deliberately cultivated in some societies.[15] On the other hand, an impressive orgasmic display and a copious ejaculate may not necessarily be unequivocal signs of fertility and potency, but simply part of the popular mythology of male sex.

To summarize these general points, then, the vasocongestion phases that accompany sexual excitation are analogous in both men and women, but they differ in their vulnerability. The male's response is more complex and therefore both more sensitive and more susceptible to sexually detractive influences than that of the female. Orgasm too is common to both sexes, but again the female orgasm — as carefully and clinically analysed by modern science — is more differentiated and consequently more ambiguous than that of the male. The orgasms of both sexes are expressed by muscular contractions of identical periodicy (0.8 second spasms), but in the woman there is no equivalent of the 'finality' of male ejaculation or the apparent necessity of a refractory period. The female response, is, therefore, more variable than that of the male.

At one level the respective responses can be interpreted in basic biochemical terms; but, important as these physical factors are, it is arguable whether they are the ultimate determinants of actual sexual expression. They govern the mechanisms of sexual activity, but they really tell us very little about *why* people act as they do in particular situations. We may be able to explain just how these mechanisms work, but — as yet — we cannot do much more than *describe* their operations. This is because many of the critical stimuli are of a psycho-social nature. The biochemistry responds — or does not respond — not only to tactile stimulation but also to a complex of psycho-social cues. It is these that give sex its 'meanings', and it is to these that we will turn next when we examine the concept of sexual 'normality' and the extrinsic facts affecting sexual malfunction.

So much then for the present theoretical state of play in studies of sexuality. What we have considered so far is an outline of the current thinking about the respective male and female response with particular reference to male sexual dysfunction. But this view is bedevilled by a certain semantic confusion (not entirely unusual in a discipline that can loosely refer to 'birth control' — strictly a term for abortion — when it really means conception control).

This confusion relates to the whole conception of 'orgasm', which is applied indiscriminately to quite separate experiences in both sexes. As we have seen, the term 'orgasm' is used to denote a particular heightening and relaxing of sexual tensions and is said to be physiologically similar in both males and females.

But is this really the case? This study maintains that the undifferentiated unisexual orgasm view is fundamentally mistaken. In so far as orgasm denotes the spasmic release of muscular tensions, then it is obviously applicable to both sexes. But the reflexive phenomenon of ejaculation in the male marks it off as something essentially different from the female experience. It is ejaculation that necessarily involves the subsequent refractory period that minimizes the male restimulation possibilities. It is, in fact, difficult to avoid the impression in the relevant texts that this renders the male somehow sexually inferior to the female in orgasmic potential. Certainly this is a line taken in popular literature that eulogizes the female sexual role (see for example Lydon, 1968).

It could however be argued that women need no refractory period *because* they do not ejaculate. That, the male experience is fundamentally distinct and altogether more significant than that of the female. Indeed, it is the contention of this study that the expression 'orgasm' for male and 'orgasm' for the female do not — and cannot — mean the same thing. In fact, it further argues that the term 'orgasm' should not be used indistinctively about both sexes, but should be reserved solely for the female experience. For the male, orgasm — tension release — plus ejaculation should possibly be thought of as a 'climax'. In the strict sense of the term, people do not have clima*xes;* the idea of a plurality of climaxes makes semantic nonsense. Women can have multiple orgasms, though men do not and perhaps — in practice — cannot. But there is nothing inherently 'superior' in this capacity. Women do not climax. The term is a misnomer when applied to the variable female experience because, by definition, a climax has a certain finality which is not easily or proximately repeatable. Any attempt to do so is an anti-climax — hence the refractory period.

This study takes a qualified 'biological' view of sex. It regards psycho-social satisfactions as important, but it also takes as unequivocal that reproduction and not recreation is the primary end of sexual activity. Sex may be intensely pleasurable, but this is simply a function of its reproductive essentiality. The male climax reflects this; all ejaculation has ostensible or actual reproductive functions. On this analysis, there is a sense in which male ejaculation is more analogous to female ovulation. This is its rough equivalent.[16] Female orgasm approximates to the male role in karezza (*coitus reservatus*), where ejaculation is controlled in such a way as to give the experience of repeated orgasm.[17]

This analysis is not intended to give pre-eminence to either sex. Obviously, the male and female have complementary reproductive roles, but their orgasmic roles, though similar, are not the same. The male climax, which is virtually inseparable from ejaculation, has a reproductive functionality, whereas the female orgasm in itself has nothing whatsoever to do with reproduction: indeed, it is perhaps no more than a welcome but adventitious by-product of the mating process.

2. The Concept of Sexual Normality

It follows from our preliminary discussion that the study of sexual impotence is vitiated by definitional nuances and problems of interpretation. One way or another, these reflect the entire spectrum of experiential possibilities. The investigation of sexual *in*adequacy automatically begs questions about sexual adequacy. What does it mean to be sexually adequate, and — more problematically — what can it mean to be sexually 'normal'? And how are these related to both sexual capacity and sexual potential?

Physical variables must be examined. We know that sexuality is affected by organic factors such as ageing and disease, and the concomitant introduction of particular drugs. But these are not the only critical influences. The fact that sexuality has a biological basis does not mean that there is a relentless uniformity about sexual expression. Sex, like every other human activity, is subject to cultural variation (see particularly Ford and Beach, 1951). The importance of socio-cultural factors may not be so marked in the matter of sexual capacities, but they are all too evident in any consideration of the differing conceptions of sexual 'normality'.

The reproductive aspects of sex have — perhaps rightly — merited considerable attention. There is an extensive literature on a variety of medical specialisms ranging from the physiology of the sex organs to the biology of pregnancy. But it is only in recent years that more intensive examinations of the *non*-reproductive aspects of sex have been made. The serious study of sexual *behaviour* really dates only from the nineteenth century. This was due *partly* to the fact that it was not until this time that the necessary investigatory techniques were being developed. But mainly it was because the moral climate was becoming more conducive to such studies. The growing desire to restrict family size and the gradual evolution and acceptance of contraceptive practices tended to shift the emphasis from the procreational to the recreational aspects of sex.

The study of sex is complicated by the kaleidoscopic variability of sexual behaviour. While the biological unity of the human species gives a basic uniformity to sexual activity, considerable variety of expression arises because of the different modes of socio-cultural adaptation. Norms are therefore difficult to assess. Statistics may not help us very much here as they only indicate 'average' patterns of behaviour, and it can be misleading to confuse the individual with the group. After any examination of group behaviour, it does not follow that inferential statements can be made about any *one* member of that group. For example, it is statistically probable that, in any group of single men between thirty-six and forty, about 22 per cent are likely to be homosexuals (Kinsey *et al.*, 1948). But this tells us nothing about the actual status of any specific individual within that group who might be almost anything from an unattached fetishist to an unlikely hermaphrodite. Complementarily, it is not advisable to extrapolate from the particular to the general. What is true for any individual cannot be extended to the group. The presence of exceptional cases — especially in sexual behaviour — can give a very distorted impression of the mean for that group.[1]

It has been suggested that assessments of 'normal' human behaviour can be made according to four criteria (see Katchadourian and Lunde, 1972, p. 151):

(1) the statistical norm: how common is this behaviour?
(2) the medical norm: is this behaviour healthy?
(3) the ethical norm: is this behaviour moral?
(4) the legal norm: is this behaviour legitimate?

Judgements made on these bases are overlapping and mutually reinforcing. What is more important is that their applications — especially in highly differentiated modern societies — can be very confusing. Statistical norms are infamously susceptible to distortion, and in practice the legal and the ethical tend to coalesce. Lastly, the medical bases of some proscribed acts may have little or no scientific validity; contrary to earlier opinions, masturbation does not even *impair* the eyesight — except perhaps in the badly placed voyeur straining at an unyielding partition.

Given the necessary reservations, therefore, about the validity of an entirely statistical approach, and the criticisms that have been levelled at particular studies (see Brecher, 1972), it is still important that we try to get some reasonable idea as to what is meant by 'sexual adequacy'.

Using orgasmic experience as a criterion, we find that, according to Kinsey's figures (Kinsey *et al.*, 1948, esp. pp. 198ff), the average sexual outlet in males in the United States from a variety of stimuli,[2] including coitus, masturbation, petting, nocturnal emission, homosexual activities and zoophilia (animal contacts), is three orgasms per week. It is obvious that there must be considerable overlapping in the criteria Kinsey uses. For instance, exactly how does one define masturbatory orgasm? Is it only autoerotic, does it follow from petting, and can it not often be included under homosexual activities?

What emerges from a comparison of the figures is that this 'average' is inflated by the more active respondents. The mode was *one* orgasm per week; this was the highest single frequency. The sample was representative of white males from the age of fifteen to eighty-five, and the frequency range extended from 0 to 29 orgasms per week with about 75 per cent of the respondents falling in the 1 to 6 orgasms per week category. Perhaps the most important single factor affecting frequency was age. The most active males were under thirty, although between twenty-six and thirty the average frequency was 2 — 3 orgasms per week (Kinsey et al., 1948), that is about the same as the mean for all males taken as a whole. Hyperactive males are in evidence in the sample; more than 7 per cent averaged 7 orgasms a week. It may be that sexual performance is at least partly governed by the circumstances that condition its expression. Some male prostitutes, for example — especially homosexual prostitutes — are able to ejaculate several times a day. And this high capacity does not appear to relate to any known socio-cultural factors (Katchadourian and Lunde, 1972, p. 163). On the other hand, there is considerable evidence of sexual restraint and actual abstinence among even the younger age groups. About 10 per cent of the fifteen-to-thirty-one years group averaged one orgasm every two weeks, and 3 per cent averaged only one orgasm every ten weeks. The orgasmic frequency of 'low-outlet' males showed a tendency to decline even further after the age of thirty-five.

It is useful to note by way of comparison that the Kinsey studies showed that, despite the theoretically greater sexual 'capacities' of the female, there was a higher incidence of sexual inactivity among them than among males. There are many social reasons that would probably account for this, but during the peak years for women, i.e. between thirty and forty, about 33 per cent had no orgasms; and about 25 per cent of the unmarried women had never had such an experience (Kinsey et al., 1953).

Statistical assessments of sex require close scrutiny, and must be subject to considerable qualifications. After all, it is impossible to gauge the quality and variety of sexual activity from figures alone. In studies such as these, the sampling methods themselves are often open to dispute (see Cochran *et al.,* 1953). But of more fundamental significance is the fact that the investigators are almost entirely at the mercy of their respondents, who sometimes appear to be either hopelessly naive or impossibly virile. Yet despite these deficiencies, the survey method has its uses, if only because it is one of the few forms of social investigation we have.

Further problems are posed by the criteria employed. The orgasm as the unit of study has serious disadvantages, if only because there is obviously a wide range of sexual activity that may not, and often does not, culminate in orgasm — especially in women. But again, with all these qualifications of orgasm as an accurate 'measure' of sexual capacity, it is still a useful indicator of customary sexual expression.

How then can we possibly decide what is 'normal'? And why do we even *want* to be normal, if normality merely connotes unexceptional behaviour?

For many, normality tends to be equated with the 'average' experience. To be below average — a sexual midget — becomes cause for concern. Deviation from the mean or what is believed to be the mean, however computed, tends to alarm people. To cast doubt upon someone's normality can be an irredeemable insult. But if 'average' is simply taken to mean 'ordinary', this may indicate an unhealthy obsession with mere mediocrity.

Escape from the tyranny of the average can be encouraging, for example, to men who are unnecessarily worried about their penis size, and to women who may be relieved to learn that at least 60 per cent of other women masturbate and indulge in unmentionable erotic fantasies (see particularly Johnson and Fretz, 1974). It can even afford some consolation to those who regard themselves as functionally inadequate. Self-doubt can be a lonely preoccupation, and is a common feature of what might be termed the Elijah syndrome.[3] To learn that there are many others like themselves can be a source of comfort, but to discover that the notion of sexual normality defies any really satisfactory definition may introduce the possibility of actual emancipation.

Of course, 'normality' usually means more than simple 'averageness', because it also implies important notions of rationality. In common usage, it suggests a kind of 'reasonableness' which itself is associated with normality. In the social sciences, however, 'rationality' has somewhat more technical connotations. More often than not it is used to denote a particular relationship between means and ends.[4] What are the most rational means for the achievement of ends which themselves may be non-rationally chosen? Relating the term rationality exclusively to means can carry with it dissonant implications of *efficiency* which are not altogether appropriate to behavioural situations. To ask about the best ways of realizing any preselected goal may have limited applications in a sexual context. If the end in question is sexual gratification, we may think in terms of the customary means, or the most suitable means, or even the most available means, but hardly in terms of the most efficient means. Efficiency suggests something almost discordantly clinical in this respect. Sexual satisfaction is essentially a non-rational objective which is arguably served by a variety of excitatory non-rational means that are not simply expeditious. It is doubtful whether insinuations of efficiency have a natural place in sexual activity; for it is just in this kind of context that their presence encourages that inhibiting sense of self-awareness that can be so detrimental to actual sexual performance.

What is considered normal must be conditioned by cultural factors, which *differ* from society to society. The given variables of sexual practice are limited — after all, there are only two sexes. But the range of experiential variations on the biologically circumscribed themes seems endless. To complicate matters even further, cultural influences are invariably bound up with moral considerations. For example, until the recent advent of the 'sex-show' Europeans were shocked at the idea of public sexual activity — even more so if it involved what we tend to regard as under-age girls. But where there are — or were — no such cultural norms, the notions of public decency or female modesty are obviously irrelevant. Consider the following incident recounted by Captain Cook concerning Polynesian mating practices in the late eighteenth century. This would simply be designated as 'savage' by modern Western standards, although it was perfectly normal for the participants:

> A young man, near six feet high, performed the rites of Venus with a little girl about eleven or twelve years of age, before several of our people, and a great number of the natives, without the least sense of being indecent or improper, but, as appeared, in perfect conformity with the custom of the place. Among the spectators were several women of superior rank . . . who may be said to have assisted in the ceremony, for they gave instructions to the girl how to perform her part, which, young as she was, she did not seem to much stand in need of. [Hawesworth, 1773, p.128]

Or to take another example, in modern Western society we tend to proscribe polygamy although historically most societies appear to have practised it. Ford and Beach (1951) in their study found that, of the 185 societies investigated, 122 were polygamous. Admittedly, most of these were primitive societies, as was the case in the earlier Murdock (1949) study of 187 societies of which only 40 were monogamous. A back-to-nature advocate might well observe that such findings simply point to the evils of education.

The business of sexual normality is riddled with inconsistencies. Take preferential marriage practices: it is possible to maintain the ideal that girls should be virgins when they marry only if the society in question has either very strong moral restrictions on pre-marital sex or allows girls to marry so young that the chances of premature defloration are reduced to a minimum. The current situation — certainly in the West — is neither quite one thing nor another. There is still a vestigial hope that girls will go to the bridal bed eager but uninitiated. But with the old moral codes fast disappearing and an upper age for marriage being retained, virgin brides are becoming distinctly scarce (see for example Schofield, 1965).

Further ambiguities can be seen in relation to illegitimacy (Rains, 1971). Even where pre-marital sex is increasingly condoned, it is still not accepted for a girl to have a child outside marriage, a norm that was also quite common in many traditional societies.[5] Unless conception control techniques are widely and rigourously employed, it is difficult to see how we can really have one without the other. Under-age sex is still — perhaps rightly — condemned, but this can never be really effective without the necessary supportive sanctions.

We are all aware that what is considered morally and culturally normal can change. We have seen this in the softening attitudes towards pre-marital sex and contraception. Yet further evidence is provided by the case of homosexuality.

Normative perceptions of homosexuality are subject to some cultural variation. It is well documented that in some pre-literate societies homosexuality has been treated with some hostility.[6] And in others, certain 'unusual' practices were once mistakenly construed as homosexual; for example, woman-to-woman marriage, a feature of the

Lovedu tribes of the Transvaal (Fortes and Evans Pritchard, 1940), was misinterpreted in this way. Strange as such practices may seem, they were in fact forms of fictive marriage contracted for politico-economic purposes, the members of these alliances usually having their own heterosexual partners. There are, of course, well attested examples of simple societies in which homosexual practices were openly acknowledged and even institutionalized, as with the Mohave Indians of Arizona (Devereux, 1937), but these are the exception rather than the rule. At a very different level of social organization we find that a number of complex pre-industrial societies were particularly tolerant towards homosexuality. Ancient Greece is commonly cited, but the situation there is often misunderstood. Homosexuality in certain forms was an established feature of the military castes of Sparta and Thebes, but pederasty certainly was specifically proscribed in Athens. The evidence suggests that for the Greeks versatility was the thing; the person who was *exclusively* homosexual was likely to be ridiculed (Flaceliere, 1973).

Attitudes to homosexuality vary, therefore, not only between societies at different periods, but also between different strata in the same societies at the same period. Certainly when we view the gradual relaxation of attitudes in our own society towards this and other issues, we can see that what passes for sexual normality is extremely variable. But this variability is *in*variably expressed within the behavioural tradition of a healthy and persistent heterosexuality. This is an inescapable norm of human society because this alone can ensure its survival — after all, the reproductive capacities of homosexual activity are severely limited.

The whole question of normality is vitiated too by the problem of paraphilia (literally, that which accompanies love). This suggests unusual and even perverted activities which are outside the ambit of 'straight' sex. The term 'paraphilia' is rather more neutral than the term 'sexual deviancy', but the connotations are much the same. Paraphilic practices can range from the sexually innovative to the sexually bizarre. Experience demonstrates that there is something for every predilection.

Paraphilia then is a very general term. If, therefore, it is taken to denote practices other than — or in addition to — 'orthodox' heterosexual activity, which normally culminates in intercourse, the boundaries of sexual deviancy become increasingly difficult to delineate. There is now ample evidence of a mushrooming market for sexual erotica. The sexual aids trade, from rainbow-coloured condoms to inflatable baby-doll surrogates, is a growing business. Similarly, the enormous increase in sexual and fetishistic fantasy in modern advertising is mirrored in the flourishing literary underworld (see particularly Freeman, 1969), which caters for specific minority interests: male homosexuality, lesbianism and transvestitism, not to mention the rubber fetishists and the bondage enthusiasts. The more one examines this sort of thing, the more astonishing is the range of deviationary tastes, apparently everything from friendly flaggellation to 'Incest — a Game for all the Family'. Preoccupation with paraphilia is undoubtedly reflected in this proliferation of cult literature and cult paraphernalia.

The real issue here is not so much whether the paraphiliac is normal — a judgement that depends almost entirely upon the perspective of the observer — but to what extent those who require supererogatory sex can be regarded as potent or impotent. If a man requires a prostitute to urinate on him before he can be fully aroused, is this really a form of sexual inadequacy? There is a well documented case of this form of sexual deviation (von Krafft-Ebing, 1899). The person in question was a man of some standing and reputation who was bitterly ashamed of his own obsession, and persistently vowed that he was never going to do it again — but to little avail. The poignancy of this example compares interestingly with some of the more ludicrous antics of occasional *Forum* correspondents (Greenwald and Greenwald, 1974), one of whom claimed that he and his wife preferred intercourse standing in a dustbin, dressed only in plastic raincoats. But the problem is still the same. Can those who indulge in such innovations be regarded as sexually adequate? And are we here thinking of males who really *need* such practices for complete sexual satisfaction, or those who simply *prefer* it for added stimulation?

Perhaps we can give more substance to this issue if we take an actual case study.

CASE A

A, the subject of this study, is in his thirties and has a wife and two children. He is a highly intelligent and well qualified academic who, to all intents and purposes, leads a perfectly ordinary life. He is susceptible to conventional forms of sexual stimulation, and capable of normal sexual intercourse, but the difference is that he prefers an *hors d'oeuvre* of mild flagellation or, at least, the pretence of flagellation. He likes his wife to tie him up before beating him as part of their love-making. There is a ritual of actual or simulated punishment, in which the wife participates, which usually involves the acting out of a fantasy in which A is both dominated and reprimanded. Sometimes other peripheral visual stimuli are included in the initial stages of sexual activity such as soft-porn 'girlie' magazines, although these have no particularly deviant emphasis. At some stage in the proceedings intercourse often takes place, but it is not an invariable feature of the ritual. A's primary concentration is on his own orgasm. His wife's satisfaction tends to be a secondary and somewhat supplementary affair. Frequently, he is finally brought to ejaculation by manual stimulation by his wife. For him, this is often a more desirable and more predictable release mechanism. Her own orgasm — a less regular occurrence — is normally achieved by masturbation, although her natural proclivity is for oral sex.

Before marriage, both partners had had relatively little sexual experience, even with each other. A's wife, whose upbringing had been unfashionably sheltered, was initially both surprised and shocked by her husband's paraphilic suggestions when they were first married. Her first instincts were completely ambivalent; she was repelled by the idea, yet she was also anxious to please him. She wanted help, to confide in someone, but in whom? At the time it seemed impossible to talk to anyone about it. She went along with what she came to regard as something of a pantomime. The ritual implements were always at hand in the bedroom, and when required she dutifully played the necessary role. As time went by, it began to seem more and more innocuous — a harmless, if rather silly, game which obviously gave someone pleasure. In the end she just settled into the routine, and accepted the situation. The abnormal gradually became esoterically normal.

When asked, A tends to interpret his own situation in terms of childhood experiences. He does not appear to have any shame or regret about these practices. They represent another kind of normality — a different *modus operandi* which he does not necessarily wish to change. What he does may be unusual, but it is certainly not unknown. In all, he seems to view his situation with an air of guiltless resignation.

Consider the general nature of these sexual activities and the modest sado-masochism involved. There is a de-emphasis on intercourse and the female orgasm; an intense concentration on the experience of ejaculation, often brought about by manual techniques; the sexual game of actual or simulated flagellation — all necessitating an almost passive role for the male. These all seem to point to a form of latent homosexuality, although this could be a simplistic — and almost glib — diagnosis of a rather complex psycho-social process. Whatever kind of reaction this sort of behaviour generates, whether it is regarded as harmless, tragic or simply disgusting, is — in one sense — rather beside the point. Clinically, these practices cannot be immoral, but they are clearly abnormal. In the strictest sociological usage they do not conform to a norm; they do not reflect the view of any kind of consensus. But for our purposes even this is not the most relevant issue. What concerns us specifically is whether men who require these hidden extras can really be said to be sexually inadequate. According to our previous definition, this would seem to be arguable. The response is adequate where the stimuli are adequate. Whether the stimuli are *appropriate* is another matter. The morality or otherwise of such practices will continue to be matters of debate. All we can say is that, in behavioural terms, they obviously work for some people some of the time.

It follows then, from our discussion so far, that there have to be accepted norms which shape our conceptions of sexual adequacy. Our notions of potency are conditioned by simple physiological imperatives. With all the liberal concessions that are appropriate to post-Kinsey society, there remain the irreducible biological minima that determine our basic judgements. There is a prevailing consensus. There are given social understandings as to what constitutes normality, and fundamentally these are governed by procreative necessity.

These assumptions about normality are related tangentially to the rather less contentious area of sexual 'capacities'. We must now ask what factors influence those capacities? What exactly induces change? Capacity implies adequacy, so can we identify just *some* of the reasons why sexual adequacy might degenerate to inadequacy?

SEX AND AGE

There are certain obvious *physical* determinants of change; these are fundamental and, in some senses, 'natural'. The least avoidable is the ageing process, which affects both men and women. In general terms, the physiological effects of ageing are fairly consistent and predictable, but there is a dearth of material on the sexual implications of growing old.[7] Again in general terms, we can say that ageing affects the intensity and regularity of sexual activity, but it is not at all clear exactly why some people are able to maintain their sexual vigour despite their years.

Among the work that has been done in this area, the Kinsey study included only a very small proportion of elderly men; a mere 106 of the 14,084 men studied were over sixty. This showed that, at sixty, three men in four were still capable of sexual intercourse.

For more recent studies, Finkle found that, among a sample of male patients between fifty-five and sixty-nine whose presenting complaints did not, in themselves, constitute impediments to sexual intercourse, 65 per cent were regarded as potent in that they claimed to have copulated at least once in the previous year. In a companion sample of men of seventy and over, by the same criterion only 34 per cent were found to be potent.[8] With comparably small samples, Pfeiffer and others (1969) have found that a very high proportion (80 per cent) of men over sixty whose health is otherwise unimpaired show a continuing interest in sexual matters, and that an only slightly smaller proportion (70 per cent) had 'regular' sexual activity.

Pfeiffer summarizes these investigations by saying that 4 out of 5 men over sixty-five who enjoy good health retain an interest in sex, while 2 out of 3 in their sixties are still sexually active. In yet a further study, Newman and Nichols (1960), with a volunteer sample of 250 men and women aged between sixty and ninety-three found — not surprisingly — that those with sexual partners were more active than those without. In this sample, of the 101 subjects *without* a sexual partner only 7 per cent were sexually active, compared with a sexually active 54 per cent of the 149 respondents who were married.

For the ageing male, the main concern is the matter of erectile adequacy. The Masters and Johnson study shows that, in the older man, erection may take longer to achieve, and although it may be possible to maintain it for comparable periods it may be more difficult to regain once it has been lost. Similarly, the climactic experience is not likely to be so intense. The time to ejaculation will be longer; the contractions will not be as vigorous, nor the ejaculate as copious as in earlier years. It follows, therefore, that refractory periods will tend to be longer, and the possibility of repeated orgasms will be appreciably diminished. What evidence there is suggests that, rather than depleting their strength, those who have pursued an active sex life in earlier years are more likely to maintain it into middle age and beyond (Katchadourian and Lunde, 1972, p. 76). Older impotent males have been very successfully treated for their condition, and often take confidence from the fact that they can control ejaculation more easily than younger men. Despite the years and the waning of natural capacities, it does seem that the key to successful sexual activity for the ageing male is adequate and appropriate stimulation (Masters and Johnson, 1966).

Although the physiological effects of ageing are, if anything, more marked in the female than in the male (Katchadourian and Lunde, 1972, pp. 76-7), evidence suggests that the sex life of the female is notably longer than that of the male. This is particularly so in the sphere of autoerotic sex. According to Kinsey, masturbation and sexual dreams continue unabated until the late fifties. Indeed, it has been argued that, where female sexual activity is reduced, this may be the result of regulation by possibly older and less active husbands (Kinsey *et al.*, 1953). This should be compared with somewhat different findings, which indicate that fewer women than men are either interested or active in their sixties. Only about 1 in 3 reports interest in sex, while a mere 1 in 5 actually has sex. And although the decline is not so marked in women as men in *advanced* age, this may be because the women have had lower interest and activity rates all their lives.[9] In general, however, it does seem that both men and women continue to retain their pleasure in the experience of orgasm, although it is important to emphasize that in this there is immense individual variation (see Pitt, 1976).

Sex and Illness

Another important factor that influences sexual normality is illness. Any debilitating condition must affect both the nature and frequency of sexual activity, and this is particularly so with male sexual performance. Most obviously this can occur after surgery, when there is usually a combination of both psychological and mechanical difficulties. These can interfere with the normal mechanisms and can inhibit erection, secretion, muscular contraction and so forth (see Watts, 1976). However, in favourable circumstances these need not be totally incapacitating, especially if those concerned are prepared to be sexually innovative. In widening their range from 'straight' intercourse to encompass a variety of manual, oral and even mechanical possibilities, a more modestly satisfying sex life might still be achieved.

What is particularly pertinent to this study are the kinds of disease that are known to be directly associated with impotence. There is a tendency in the literature to minimize these organic problems. Instead, the stress is put — perhaps rightly — on presumed psychological causes. These do appear to be much more common, but physical factors should not be overlooked. A presenting patient complaining of impotence should ensure that some cursory examination or at least inquiry is made, if only to eliminate these organic possibilities before any further therapy is attempted. Similarly, it is equally important to distinguish between diseases that are *directly* related to impotence and those that are merely sexually inhibiting.

There is a general category of conditions in which intercourse and possibly other kinds of sexual activity could prove painful. This could include arthritis, hernias and even extreme obesity. Primarily, there are certain conditions of the sexual organs themselves which occasion extreme discomfort. These may either prevent or inhibit stimulation and response, and might range from an easily rectifiable tight foreskin to more serious local infections, including sexually transmitted (venereal) diseases such as gonorrhoea or advanced syphilis. But they could also include the increasingly common 'nuisance' infections, such as thrush and trichomonas, which are most common in women but can be transferred to the male. These can be extremely persistent and frustrating. Despite the ritual of unending applications of anti-fungoidal preparations, the danger of re-infection is always present.

In a somewhat different category come diseases that require surgery or conditions where some kind of surgical operation has already been carried out. Abdominal or bowel resections, and particularly operations either required or performed to remove tumours from the prostate, a relatively common condition in ageing males, can all have direct effects on sexual potency.

Neurological disorders, especially those that affect the spinal cord, will also be directly injurious to the male sexual response. Multiple sclerosis is a prime example, but what is probably less well known is that impairment of the nervous system with accompanying impotence frequently results from diabetes. Endocrine (glandular) and liver disorders such as hepatitis tend to affect androgen (male hormone) levels, which in turn may affect sexuality. And cardio-vascular diseases can impair erectile responses by interference with the penile blood supply (Kaplan, 1974, pp. 75-85).

SEX AND DRUGS

The deleterious effects of particular drugs on male sexuality have probably been both understated and underreported. Some drugs act directly on the brain, others on the peripheral nerve centres. As such they can affect all aspects of sexual response: erection, emission, and even the sex drive itself. It is well known, for example, that if the level of the male hormone testosterone is reduced, the effect can be tantamount to a kind of chemical castration.[10] Many factors may influence testosterone levels. They may be low because of illness, but they can also be reduced by deliberate medication. If, for example, counter-acting estrogenic (female hormone) preparations are administered — as they often are for certain urological disorders — the side-effects can produce the inability to have an erection and perhaps loss of libido, i.e. the desire for and interest in normal sexual activity (Kaplan, 1974, pp. 50-1).

Drugs that can impair sexual activity are frequently prescribed by the most well-meaning physicians for a whole variety of conditions. And these are quite apart from those other categories of drugs popularly distinguished as 'hard drugs' and 'soft drugs' — particularly tobacco and alcohol — with which society, or sections of it, insists on undermining its health. Contrary to popular myth, neither these nor any other known drug can definitely be shown to *increase* sexual response or enjoyment, although some may *enhance* it under certain conditions. The stimulus effect of certain experimental drugs[11] has still to be decisively demonstrated (see Beaumont, 1976). As yet, the search for the all-purpose aphrodisiac is little more than a priapic dream. But, predictably, the 'trade' is working on it.

The unwanted sexual side-effects of drugs are more clearly understood and obviously more readily detected in the male than in the female. Any disturbance in the male sexual response is easier to identify and substantiate. Failed erection and retarded ejaculation are not particularly easy to hide, whereas inability to lubricate in the female is — as we have seen — a matter of some ambiguity.

For convenience, drugs and their sexual side-effects can be simply classified as those that primarily affect libido or erection or ejaculation (Beaumont, 1974), although it should be emphasized that these categories are not mutually exclusive.

Libido

The male sex drive can be adversely affected by a number of drugs which are prescribed for otherwise good medical reasons. But the assessment of their specific effects is sometimes difficult because other variables creep into the equation. If particular drugs are being taken to alleviate the symptoms of any specific condition, general depression over that condition may well inhibit sexuality anyway. In this case the drugs concerned, whose chemical action may in fact be entirely neutral, could be mistakenly thought to have affected sexual desire. Anti-depressant, anti-anxiety and anti-psychotic drugs can all indirectly improve sexual functioning. When the depression itself is effectively relieved, the patient may recover some semblance of libidal normality. Yet in other circumstances, a depressed person could be taking anti-depressant drugs that might well *increase* his depression simply because the drugs, acting upon the autonomic system, suppressed libido and thus gave rise to further anxieties. There is the parallel argument that drugs which can cause loss of libido can indirectly act as anti-depressants. The ongoing debate about the effects of oral contraceptives is a case in point. The problem is not yet resolved, but it *may* be that the 'pill' actually decreases sexual desire, but this is offset by the woman's relief at having certain protection against unwanted or unplanned pregnancies.

Most notoriously and perhaps most commonly, it is sedatives of various kinds that can have detrimental effects on sex drive. Hypnotic and barbiturate drugs frequently prescribed as sleeping tablets can cause problems of this kind, as also can alcohol, which is traditionally reputed to both increase desire but reduce performance.[12] Narcotics, which are customarily used as pain-killers, also act upon the central nervous system. Even in their milder analgesic forms, such as codeine, they can have almost imperceptibly deleterious effects.

Anti-androgens too, as we have already seen, have their problems. Estrogen preparations, which are sometimes given in cases of prostate cancer, and cortisone, which is commonly prescribed especially for allergic and orthopaedic conditions, must also be included among those drugs that may adversely affect sexual desire. But again, it must be emphasized that the conditions for which they are prescribed could well involve such distress that it would be virtually impossible to say if the drugs alone were the sufficient cause of euthemic deficiency.[13]

Erection

The complex mechanism of erection is sensitive to many psycho-social factors. Sometimes these influences are quite incalculable. Therefore it is important to establish, where possible, whether particular instances of erectile impotence are — or might be — the result of organic or psychological factors before impatiently ascribing them to drug therapy. However, it is scientifically attested that erection is susceptible to the action of a variety of chemical agents. Again, some anti-depressants and certain amine inhibitors (the MAO group of drugs), which may be prescribed, among other things, for migraine, can impair erection if taken in sufficient doses. Also sometimes used in the treatment of migraine are the ganglion-blocking drugs (beta-blockers) which are probably more commonly employed for the alleviation of hyper-tension.[14] These are known to have corresponding effects on sexual performance, although, given the crippling effects of such afflictions as migraine, it must be arguable that the risk is worth it. Anti-adrenergic drugs which block the adrenergic nerves are also used for hypertension and certain vascular disorders, and can have similar deleterious effects including additional ejaculatory problems. This group of drugs includes ergot compounds, which are used extensively in the treatment of migraine, significantly as a prophylactic which has to be taken in regular doses on a more-or-less permanent basis.

Ejaculation

Ejaculatory problems can be roughly divided into those concerned with retarded ejaculation, and those involving 'dry' ejaculation. Again the most frequently cited drugs are the anti-adrenergic group used primarily for hypertension, and the psychotropic drugs used to combat anxiety or depression and which may actually affect the sperm count

(Beaumont, 1976, p. 333). Ejaculatory difficulties have also been reported — though rather infrequently — in connection with the MAO group (monoamine oxidase inhibitors). Perhaps the most serious effects have been attributed to antipsychotic drugs which are most notably used in the treatment of schizophrenia. It is hypothesized that these may cause the semen to empty into the bladder, thus giving a 'dry' ejaculation.[15]

Some drugs may have the ambiguous effect of both enhancing *and* inhibiting sexual performance. These are often referred to as stimulants, but there is a sense in which this is something of a misnomer. The most common of these, alcohol, taken in small doses can act indirectly as a mild stimulant by reducing anxiety and 'releasing' inhibitions. It does not act directly on the sex centres. In fact, it is a brain depressant, and in large doses has anaesthetizing effects, impairing both sexual performance and cognitive functions (Lemere and Smith, 1973). As we have noted, barbiturates and hypnotic drugs have similar behavioural effects. Cocaine and amphetamine users claim increased sexual pleasure at certain dose levels. But both are highly addictive, and the evidence suggests that users become increasingly more interested in the drug than in the sexual side-effects that it produces. Even more serious reservations would apply to heroin, *and* to methadone, which is sometimes given to heroin addicts in order to wean them away from their cravings for the drug. These narcotics depress the central nervous system and markedly reduce both sexual interest and capacity.

The question of LSD and marijuana presents somewhat different problems. Both are hallucinogenic drugs which act on the central nervous system, but their effects vary considerably. LSD-users often report that their sexual activity has a 'detached' quality (Kaplan, 1974, pp. 89-90), it is 'interesting' rather than exciting — which must be a highly subjective evaluation. Again, there tends to be a preoccupying involvement with the drug and the *range* of 'experience' that it brings rather than any specific enhancement of sexuality. In all this, there are strong qualitative overtones. Users claim new dimensions of consciousness; the purely exotic is seen as superior to the merely erotic; inner mental exploration is held to transcend the prosaicism of mere physical expression.

Quite a lot of research has been done, especially in the United States, on the impact of marijuana on sexuality. The general conclusions vary somewhat in emphasis, and are understandably coloured by tacit social norms which prescribe the differential expectations of sexual behaviour for males and females. This is reflected in some of the literature (see for example Kolansky and Moore, 1971). Female users are said to be 'promiscuous' while males are said to be sexually overactive. The implication in some studies is that the drug is taken in order to compensate for known or anticipated 'sexual incompetence'.[16] In general, the effects of the drug are partly conditioned by the conventions of the user's sub-culture. It follows, therefore, that they are also intensely subjective. Several studies have shown that the majority of respondents report enhanced sexual appetite and sexual pleasure while 'high' on marijuana.[17] This is, perhaps surprisingly, more the case with habitual users than with infrequent users. Respondents speak of heightened sensitivity and the impression that the sex act lasts longer; objectively, this may be an illusion.

Marijuana use tends to go with a particular life style in which increased sexual activity plays a part. It is associated, particularly in the United States, with counter-culture ideologies which are often anti-intellectual as well as anti-authoritarian in orientation. Behaviour involving spontaneity, immediacy and emotional engagement may come to be regarded as highly desirable, while activities demanding precision, technical mastery and sustained effort may be denigrated as unrewarding. In a sense, sex is essentially a non-rational activity which is barely enhanced by cerebral reflection. Hence the sometimes excessive and chronic habituation to a variety of drugs that transitionally heighten the sexual experience, but which can eventually lead to dispiriting forms of sexual impotence (Peterson, 1974, p. 164).

To summarize: the matter of sexual capacities needs considerable qualification. A variety of factors, both physical and biochemical, can induce changes which often can either be rectified or their effects ameliorated. Even more problematical is the question of sexual normality that is vitiated by definitional arguments and substantive complexities. However, the general contention of this thesis is that, assuming there is no biochemical abnormality, men will respond sexually given adequate and appropriate stimulation. Drugs and illness can obviously impair sexual efficiency. They can affect normal performance *levels* but not — in the main — basic behavioural normality. The response itself can be educated and even conditioned. Socialization processes will undoubtedly influence the ways in which it is directed, but they can only modify an elemental sexuality. The *kinds* of things that induce sexual desire and, therefore, sexual response are achieved by psycho-cultural factors and are merely operationalized by the chemistry. Erection may be produced by the autonomic nervous system, but in normal sexual practice it is the recognition and interpretation of the requisite signals that actually triggers the response. These signals can be visual or olfactory, tactile or purely intellectual. In practice, it will be an amalgam of these — the 'mix' may not really matter. It is the combination of stimulus and response, not the transmission mechanisms themselves, that will ultimately determine a man's potency or impotency.

3. The Incidence of Impotence I: Some Comparative and Historical Perspectives

It is believed that there is an increasing incidence of sexual dysfunction — particularly male impotence — in Western society (Parr, 1975). This cannot, of course, be proved, but the persistent reiteration of such themes in the media at least suggests heightened anxieties.

It should be made quite clear at the outset of this phase of the discussion that the *actual* incidence of impotence is quite impossible to determine. If the iceberg theory of submerged potential response operates anywhere, it is surely in the area of sexual dysfunction. With all the much-applauded openness about sex, people are not prepared to broadcast their operational shortcomings. In fact, the freer sexual climate probably inhibits as much as it inspires. The modern stress on performance levels does not exactly encourage humiliating admissions of sexual incompetence. Therapists may attract hesitant inquirers, but straight researchers — who carry less conviction and absolutely no authority — have a more demanding task. Nobody wants to come forward. As one sympathetic health official unwittingly put it, 'Impotent males? Hm . . . they're very difficult to get hold of'.

The general incidence of impotence can only be hazardously guessed from certain modern trends. It is well established, for example, that there has been an increase in the practice of sex therapy. There is a small but growing band of professionals whose activities are receiving approved comment in the popular press. The Marriage Guidance Council has also set up sex therapy clinics which they expect to be the first of many to bring 'new hope for thousands of unhappy couples' ('Look-out', 1977). The probability of increased incidence can also be inferred from articles, letters to the press, magazine advice columns and so on. We are confidently informed that 'the most embarrassing question for a man is not "How much do you earn?" but "How good are you in bed?" ' (Heeming, 1977). Another probing columnist asks, 'Are you a good enough lover?' (Carr, 1977). This presumably reflects not only a perennial interest in sexual matters, but possibly also a growing concern about them. It would be easy to dismiss this sort of thing as mere tit-bits for the jaded Sunday morning palate, a kind of pseudo-therapy for the afflicted and a source of smug reassurance for the sexually athletic. But it could also express a deep underlying uncertainty. The reader must be tempted to ask, 'Can it happen to me?' And the substance of the articles will leave him with no iron-clad guarantees. He can only take comfort from a little historicist optimism and hope that the successful patterns of the past can be confidently repeated in the future.

The increasing attention that is obviously being given to matters of this kind inevitably raises the question of the extent to which impotence is essentially a condition of modern society. Is modern man not as sexually competent as his earlier, less cultured counterpart, or is he just more preoccupied with sexual concerns and implicit sexual comparisons? And how are these issues related?

The anthropologist, Bronislau Malinowski (1953, pp. 53-4), suggested that primitives exhibit an absence of sexual inhibitions. In his study of Melanesians he maintains that chastity is unknown among the natives, who are introduced to the intricacies of sex at an early age. Even in a society where women often initiate sexual activities, men did not appear to experience sexual neuroses. What anxieties they had seemed to derive from restraints on their sexuality rather than from expectational fears. Their dreams betrayed no doubts about impotence relating to female demands. If anything, their worries were of a different order — that there were certain institutional constraints which curbed completely free sexual expression (Malinowski, 1927, pp. 195-6). But these conclusions should be compared with those deriving from other primitive societies where there was an insistence on premarital chastity, and where certain sexual fears were clearly expressed. For example, among the Ambo of Northern Rhodesia youths were discouraged from marrying a fully mature woman 'lest she overcome him and he fails in coitus' (Stefaniszyn, 1964, pp. 99-100). Instead, he was enjoined to fortify himself with medicines to improve his sexual organs and then marry a young underdeveloped girl. There is an oblique reflection of similar attitudes in monographs from the Solomon Islands. But there it was treated as a joke if in play a boy tried to copulate before his penis could harden (Oliver, 1955, p. 72).

Some anxieties about impotence certainly existed in the primitive world. Among the Plateau Tonga, a newly married woman could legitimately leave her husband if he was sexually inadequate (Colson, 1951, p. 164). In Swazi society, if a husband proved to be impotent his brother might surreptitiously take on the task of impregnating the wife to give the husband children, although discovery of the act might cause the husband to commit suicide (Marwick, 1940, p. 136). Zulu doctors had specific remedies for impotence, but — as far as can be judged — they were not very much in evidence. A.T. Bryant (1949,

p. 637) insisted that the Zulu were 'more lastingly virile' than Europeans, and that among them impotence was rare except for 'organic derangement' brought about by white man's diseases. In general, then, the monographs say little or nothing about the incidence of impotence in primitive society. It obviously occurred, but it does not appear to have been a besetting or widespread problem. Where it is mentioned, it is not unusual to find that it is related to elderly males — possibly chiefs — who were anxious about the succession. Ethnographic and historical studies are not always clear on such matters; it is often a case of arriving at inferential conclusions from more inclusive practices. Again, in traditional Zulu society an old man with a young wife might invite a young warrior to mate with her so that any children born of that union could be reared in *his* name (Forde and Radcliffe-Brown, 1950). In this case, it would be reasonable to assume that the elderly husband was impotent, but this tells us almost nothing about the incidence of impotency among the Zulu, or whether it had more general applications in the lower age ranges. Such practices merely indicate that impotence occurred where it was to be most expected — in elderly males — and that this society had informal 'remedies' for perpetuating its patrilineal system.

It could be argued that the premium that was put upon bridal virginity in both tribal and complex societies may spring indirectly from male impotency fears. Ostensibly, virgin brides were often regarded as more desirable simply because they were innocent and unsullied. In traditional Sri Lanka (Ceylon) a white cloth was spread on the marriage bed to be stained when the bride's hyman was ruptured. This was inspected by the bride's dhobi woman, and if all was well it was announced to a waiting household; later, when the bride's parents were duly informed, there followed all the appropriate celebrations (Ryan,1958,p.75). In the Chinese tradition, the bride's 'nether garment' was sent to the bridegroom's mother, and in accordance with Cantonese custom a pig was sent to the bride's mother after the marriage had been consummated. If the pig was intact there was no cause for alarm, but if it was mutilated the bride's virginity was in question (Freedman, 1957, p. 137). In some societies the bridegroom's assurances about his bride's virginity were regarded as sufficient, and possibly a certain amount of covering up was done to protect reputations (Lang, 1946, p. 126). In other societies penalties could be severe. In Japanese society, a bride whose chastity was questioned was supposed to strangle herself with her own sash (Mace and Mace, 1960, pp. 167-8). Some Hindus imposed fines for misrepresenting a girl as a virgin, although others held that male contact with an unruptured hymen might damage the penis for ever.[1] But this appears to be a somewhat exceptional view.

It may be that the known desirability for virgins was related to the virtual certainty that they were free from venereal disease. Syphilis was almost certainly unknown in the Old World before the fifteenth century. Modern scholarship favours the view that it was brought back from the Americas by the sailors of Columbus, although the argument still continues (see Siegfried, 1965). But there are few doubts about gonorrhea, with which the ancients seem to have been quite well acquainted. It follows, therefore, that one guarantee of immunity from disease was for a man to marry a virgin.

Virgin brides were undoubtedly also in demand where succession issues were at stake. Paternity has always been an important question where legal inheritance is concerned. On such matters there must be no ambiguities. Again, virginity in the female offered the best possibilities.

But what is more pertinent to the present study is the possibility that the premium put upon virgin brides derived, and perhaps still derives, from a different kind of uncertainty — that of male sexual insecurity. Experienced women can make comparisons, and some men undoubtedly fear that their sexual performance is going to be compared unfavourably with that of others. The one sure method of obviating this possibility was by marriage to a virgin. In this way no invidious comparisons could be made. Male sexual inadequacy would presumably go undetected where no norms of performance had been established. Virgin brides, therefore, provided a certain measure of insurance against the possibilities of coital anxiety. But whether this can be *directly* related to impotence as such is still very much an open question.

It is somewhat parenthetical to the general discussion, but nevertheless interesting, that the myths of traditional societies are replete with sexual allusions. They recount diversions and perversions of every shape and variety, from incest[2] to bestiality;[3] from incredible stories of the Mesopotamian Enki, who 'causes his phallus to water the dikes' (Kirk, 1976, p. 95), to the Egyptian sky-god Atum, who creates his divine companions by masturbatory techniques (Carlton, 1977, p. 210). Many of these stories are almost aggressively phallic; there is scarcely a hint about impotence. If anything, they revel in hypersexuality; undersexed gods just do not seem to be part of the ancient cosmos.[4]

Linked with myth is what might be loosely termed 'sex magic', which was a common practice in several traditional societies. These rituals were part of many ancient religions and express refluent sexual themes; for example the sacred marriage of the Babylonians, in which intercourse was believed to have both an ecological as well as a ritual significance (see Contenau, 1969); or the mandatory coitus after combat of the Zulu warrior, ambiguously called 'the wiping of the spear', who, having presumably killed the enemy was now expunging the deed in an ostensible act of procreation (see Morris, 1968). This 'postscript' to battle could be performed almost casually with any suitable available woman, who was under an equal obligation to participate in the ritual.

Phenomena such as these provide interesting insights into the history and variety of sexual practice. They also indicate the importance of ritual and ideological imperatives. But they are only indirectly relevant to problems of sexual dysfunction. If anything, they tend to stress fertility rather than potency. In all these myths and acts, potency is assumed and, by implication, admired. Both the adequacy and acceptibility of sexual expression appear to be taken for granted.

In briefly reviewing the subject of potency historically and comparatively, it is interesting to see that it is occasionally treated as a specific problem in classical and other early literature. These references are relatively rare, but are perhaps worth noting if only for the rather bizarre remedies that were sometimes prescribed. In ancient Mesopotamia it was advocated that incantations might play a useful role in sexual activity. These were recited by women to men to give them extra stimulation. If there were erectile difficulties, the recommendation was to rub the penis with puru-oil mixed with pulverized metal particles. This, like other ancient treatments, sounds extremely uncomfortable but was presumably designed to give added friction (Biggs, 1967). The Indian Vedas similarly esteem magico-ritual incantations, although in this case there is the warning that harmful spells can make men impotent.[5]

A number of ancient authors, including Pliny, Theophrastus and Dioscorides, mention impotency in connection with Greek society (see particularly Licht, 1932). Pliny, for example, in *Historia Naturalis* classifies a number of plants as responsible agents. Agnus causes sexual weakness; eating 'boy-cabbage' dry can result in a diminished sexual impulse (xxiv 59/95 xxvii 65), although taken fresh with goat's milk can actually excite the sexual impulse. Similarly, if the plant speoluta was laid under a man it made him impotent (xxi 184), and anyone who 'drinks of sea-roses' (i.e. water-lilies) must pay for it by being impotent for twelve days (xxv 75). Pliny also assures us that the ashes of the plant brya mixed with the urine of an ox can cause impotence, and adds that some magicians can effect the same condition if it is mixed with the urine of a eunuch (xxiv 72). If males urinated where a dog had already done so, impotence ensued (xxix 102, 143), and — rather more unlikely — the same plight befell those who were daubed with mouse-dung (xxviii 262). Both Clement of Alexandria (*Stromata,* vii 4.843) and Horace (*Satires,* i 8.30) evidently echo a long-held superstition when they insist that some people had secret powers, including the ability to make others impotent, and this they ascribed to the use of woollen thread.

Ancient authors included among their folk knowledge remedies for infertility and means of averting the 'evil eye', besides a medley of love-potions and aphrodisiacs. Some of these are relatively modest. Aristophanes, the Greek comic playwright, suggests lentils, especially for the old,[6] others recommend onions to improve both desire and performance.[7] More colourful prophylactics range from the pith of the branch of a pomegranate tree to the wearing of the right testicle of an ass as a bracelet (Pliny, xxviii 261).

Similar anxieties are also reflected in Roman literature. The poet Horace, in anticipating the inadequacies of old age, says plaintively that:

> graceful youth will soon vanish . . . [and]
> drowsy and wrinkled age will deaden
> our wanton loves. [*Odes,* ii 11]

Ovid, too, in one of his poems imagines himself in the role of an impotent man (Amores, iii 7), and, in one of the most erotic pieces of classical literature, (*Satyricon*), Petronius describes impotence in some detail. As a remedy, not only does he prescribe certain foods and the invocation of the appropriate deities; he also advises the patient to introduce a phallus into his anus which has previously been smeared with a concoction of oil, pepper and nettleseed. This treatment is to be duly supplemented with a token scourging of the offending genitals with a bunch of green nettles. Whether this represents current practice, or whether — more likely — it is a product of Petronius' detumescent daydreams, it is difficult to know. Perhaps the advice that comes closest to that of modern therapy is that given by Theodorus Priscianus in the fourth century AD. As a cure for impotence, he suggests that the patient should be 'surrounded by beautiful girls or boys; also give him books to read which stimulate lust and in which love-stories are insinuatingly treated' (Licht, 1932, p. 514).

The fear of sexual impotency has been a recurring theme in certain varieties of 'love' literature through the ages. Shaykh Nefzawi, the author of *The Perfumed Garden,* had his own special recipe for stimulating an erection. He suggested that the flaccid organ would respond if the subject ate an unwholesome mixture of garlic, honey, cinnamon, hellebore, nutmeg and cardamoms together with syrup of vinegar, peppers and sparrows' tongues.

At the same time the desirability of male potency has been continually reiterated in erotic literature. There are constant reminders in writings from traditional societies of the delights of sexual congress. In Islamic lore, Muhammed's reputation is enhanced by unsubstantiated stories of virility even in his old age (Inglis, 1974). Later folk tales are still more exaggerated, until we have hyperbolic accounts in *A Thousand and One Nights* of a character who possesses forty women thirty times each in one night. Fantasies these may be, but almost certainly fantasies that reflect overt desires and perhaps latent fears.

In such sexually oriented societies as traditional India and China, very positive attitudes were both inculcated and expressed. Hindu mythology taught that sex was of divine origin; even creation itself was seen in sexual terms. In the Indian tradition there are literally hundreds of manuals extolling the virtues of sexual activity and cataloguing the various ways in which it can be enjoyed.[8] The genitalia and other erogenous zones were regarded as sacred, and their representations were often used symbolically in worship.[9] The question of potency was particularly relevant, and the more esoteric sex cults cultivated the ritual of *coitus reservatus* so as to delay and even avoid ejaculation, so that the semen would be 'transmitted to the brain'.[10] This presumably preserved the devotees' strength and enabled them to repeat the act with greater frequency.

Very similar ideas were also current in ancient China, where it was believed that if the male could retain his semen it also helped to preserve his youth.[11] In fact, Taoists taught a technique that involved exerting pressure on the urethra between the scrotum and the anus at the moment of ejaculation in order to preserve the semen. In reality, it was merely diverted to the bladder, but an elementary physiology held that it had actually been retained and could revivify the 'upper parts' of the body. Apparently contrary to this was the view that potency could be developed by persistent practice. Some Taoists held that 'the ways of sex' helped to cultivate the 'life-force', but that this could best be achieved by intercourse with many women. This kept men young in both action and appearance (van Gulik, 1970, p. 24). There is an obvious relationship between potency and polygamy, where a man must presumably be capable of satisfying a plurality of women. In traditional societies such capacities were often associated with rulers, who commanded large numbers of wives, consorts and concubines. In China, for example, we find that three was the magic number of male potency, and multiples of three indicated superabundant potency, the highest of which represented the royal potential (van Gulik,

1970, pp. 16-17). In all this, there seems to have been an underlying fear that women might learn the secret ways of the manuals, so in the Chinese tradition little is said about female sexual techniques although the masculine ones are carefully and minutely described (Bullough, 1976, p. 290).

On the reverse side, we find some concern for conditions of sexual deprivation. This applies particularly to eunuchs, although even these — depending to some extent on their degree of genital disability[12] — were sometimes employed for sexual purposes. This might be as 'passives' for anal homosexuality or for active oral-genital purposes, as in India. Some eunuchs were found desirable by harem women, because they were still capable of intercourse but not of impregnation (cf. *A Thousand and One Nights*).

The desire for potency and the corresponding anxiety about impotency can be seen in the widespread use of artificial devices for sexual purposes. Some were crudely or carefully fashioned substitutes, either artificial penises or vaginas, which were probably used ritualistically as well as privately. Others were what we would now term 'aids', that is, performance-enhancing devices or contraptions which were designed either to give extra pleasure or to make up for some known or assumed deficiency. Marginally related to such concerns was the practice of sexual cursing. It was believed by some (Bullough, 1976, pp. 246-7) that spells could be cast that induced impotency in an enemy or a sexual rival. Obviously, those who experienced impotence could comfort themselves by the knowledge that their problems were really the responsibility of others who wished them harm.

All these beliefs and practices show a perennial concern with the issues of potency and impotency, and of an implicit antagonism between the sexes. What is particularly interesting is that, in those traditional societies where there was an explicit recognition of the female sexual role and where female sexuality was actively encouraged, e.g.

in ancient China and especially India, there does not seem to have been an increasing incidence of male impotence. According to modern Women's Liberation theory, men retreat when women discover their own sexual potential. On this analysis, they should have been sadly afflicted societies, but the evidence — such as it is — suggests quite the opposite. They appear to have been vigorously and unashamedly potent — one might almost say, sexually chauvinistic.

To modern man, many of the ideas that are associated with traditional societies seem preposterous even if we appreciate some of the underlying problems that generated them. It is obvious that, in trying to discern the 'reasons' for impotency, many early writers show considerable sophistication while others inevitably betray their inability to handle such matters, because they highlight the difficulties that pre-scientific men had in trying to identify the causes of things. Their diagnoses rest upon the uncertainties of folklore and superstition, and the remedies they propose show clearly their limited capacities for empirical verification.

In defence of these extremities, it is perhaps worth reiterating that in this whole area of diagnosis and remedial treatment we still have our own problems. Cures, alleviatives and palliatives of every variety are still with us: powdered Rhino horn, 'sex water' from a spring in Bosnia, even costly animal implantations — a form of 'cellular therapy' involving buttock injections of animal foetuses in solution — are recommended for the reactivation of sexual vigour. There is no sure evidence of actual sexual rejuvenation, although patients sometimes claim that they feel better for the treatment (Inglis, 1974). So even today we can only advance plausible causal hypotheses to account for the condition. These, admittedly, have more respectable experimental foundations, and therefore inspire some therapeutic confidence. But *understanding* the problem is another question altogether. Modern clinical techniques may validate certain behavioural theories of treatment, but the matter of satisfactory *explanations* remains persistently elusive.

4. The Incidence of Impotence II: The Current Situation

Information about the nature and incidence of impotence in modern society comes from seven main sources:

(1) the popular press: in the form of occasional articles and the unwearying recital of court cases with newsworthy sexual overtones;

(2) women's magazines: again in articles, but particularly as an oft-repeated theme of the ubiquitous problem-page. Also in magazine-type radio programmes, such as 'Woman's Hour';

(3) 'confidence' magazines of the *Forum* variety whose letter/advice columns constitute a kind of thinking-man's graffiti;

(4) feminist literature: in its more esoteric forms this could almost be an incitement to impotence. The feminist jubilation at the 'fall' of the male would appear to herald the new age of Amazonian supremacy (see for example Mitchell, 1973);

(5) sex therapists: these are often psychiatrists or doctors who may be in general practice at hospitals but who also run public or private clinics. Some of their findings are to be found in highly specialized journals which are occasionally collated and published as 'Readers';[1]

(6) specialized agencies: such as the Family Planning Association, National Marriage Guidance Council, etc.;
(7) specialized research: this of necessity is small-scale and is conducted with limited resources and therefore limited objectives.

The present study attempts to combine an appraisal of both the popular and the hearsay with information taken from specialist writers. But it also includes additional material based on personal research which may act as a salutary corrective to the ambiguous impressions derived from secondary sources.

Media treatment of sexual dysfunction is certainly increasing. Whether this merely reflects the new openness about sex or whether it should be seen as something of a barometer of social concern is difficult to know. Direct coverage in the popular press is still somewhat sporadic, but exploratory articles that pose or illuminate sexual problems appear to be a regular feature of some high-circulation magazines. The snag is that, although these can — and perhaps do — have a therapeutic function, they can also reinforce suspicions of sexual inadequacy.

Not unexpectedly, these articles have a mild but marketable sensationalism, yet on the whole they are generally helpful and consolatory.[2] Sexual problems are seen to derive mainly from increased — and sometimes intolerable — social pressures. The high pace and even higher expectations of modern living are said to result in fatigue and frustration which are fatal to sexual intentions. Consequently, many articles stress the need to get back to basics. Sexual re-education is the panacea. Readers are enjoined to try to avoid unnecessary tensions, to make time for relaxation, and to give themselves the opportunity to rediscover the pleasures of sexuality. This is surely reflected in the explicit orientations of much modern advertising.

The stress on leisure pursuits, from the escapist acceptability of alcohol to the getaway romanticism of overseas vacations, often contains implicit sexual motivations. The need to relax, to unwind, to treat oneself to a night out, a good meal or a good holiday can conceal a lightly disguised sexual promise. There are, of course, cautionary tales which warn the reader that sex is hardly a seasonal indulgence, and that any solutions must be firmly based upon the recognition of everyday realities. Most people spend most of their time in a highly routinized world of mundane tasks. Research shows that some people's sex lives do improve significantly when they are on holiday, or when they are away from the children; non-orgasmic women sometimes become orgasmic, and some men recover their sex drive. Perhaps this is because holidays are the socially approved times for people to do what they want to *when they feel like doing it* — and spontaneity is of the essence in sexuality. But sufficient time plus sufficient energy does not equal satisfactory sex (see Johnson and Masters, 1975). Similarly, improved techniques, although useful, do not provide a sufficient answer. Important as all these things are, there are other factors that must enter the equation. Perhaps there is no ultimate solution to any particular sexual problem, but there are *strategies* that can be employed, and a strategy can be regarded as truly useful only if it is effective in everyday contexts.

The treatment of sexual dysfunction in women's magazines is not invariably trivial. In general, it is sympathetic and informed, but it also tends to be guarded and — naturally — female-oriented. In the advice columns, it is still possible to be assailed by the 'I'm fourteen-but-have-never-had-a-boyfriend,-what-shall-I-do? type of correspondence, but there are other letters which obviously indicate more serious problems, for example a request for help from a woman who cannot understand why, after many years of marriage, 'relations have ceased'. Though not explicitly stated, the allusion is to some indifference or inability on the part of the husband — at least, this is certainly assumed in the printed reply (Marryat, 1977b). Or there is the less guarded respondent who asks for advice because she wants to marry a widower of sixty who 'says he is unable to make love' even though he had been given chemical treatment by his doctor. The patient's subsequent readiness not to waste the good lady's life sounds less like chivalry than the well-known strategic withdrawal, but this does not preclude the possibility of genuine potency problems (Marryat, 1977a). Rather more poignant is the case where an older wife complains that her 'sex life has almost vanished'. She is convinced that her younger husband masturbates, and has attributed his waning enthusiasm for love-making to 'age and general worries over money and so on'. The respondent is assured that she is not 'to blame' (even though her letter suggests it), but this can be little more than a diplomatic reply. It is a reasonable inference that she suspects that she is no longer so attractive to her husband and that this is the primary explanation for his indifference. She may well be right, but the advice she is given dare not confirm it, as she obviously does not want to admit it even to herself (Marryat, 1976b). In some cases it is the men who make the excuses where it is evident that sex has become 'too much trouble', but few seem prepared to take expert advice or consult a doctor (Marryat, 1976a). This may be because of a natural reluctance to admit such problems even to a specialist; on the other hand, it may be that in many cases the answer is all too simple. The gut-reaction has gone, and it has gone because, for a variety of reasons, the woman just does not excite as she once did. Women hardly wish to recognize this as a determinative factor, but it has some support from recent research. The female body has been termed 'nature's spark-plug of male libido and potency', but Dr Wolbarst, the American specialist, maintains that 'there is no sexual deadener like the female. A plump, slatternly wife is a powerful sexual inhibitor, a great non-stimulus' (Inglis, 1974) — a view that is undoubtedly encouraged by the renewed emphasis upon the lubricious exposure of the human form and youthful desirability.

Sexual problems must presumably lie behind the faithful rehearsal of Women's Liberation themes in the more literate sections of the Sunday press. Renate Olins, executive information officer of the London Marriage Guidance Council, argues that problems arise because men and women are adjusting to new social roles. Women are now less submissive and are under pressure from the media to demand more in the bedroom. But how much can they demand? Are they doomed to disappointment because they have over-estimated the male sexual appetite? Mrs Olins takes the view that until now many men have successfully concealed their sexual inadequacies. They have hidden behind the adage that marriage is the price men pay for sex, and sex is the price women pay for marriage.

> This has . . . enabled them to hide behind any lack of sexual desire that they might have had. If they wanted sex every night, then they were wonderful virile guys. If they wanted it once a month, they were wonderful considerate husbands who didn't trouble their wives too much. Either way they won. Now, as in every other aspect of life, they are having to live on a much more equal footing. It is very painful for many of them. [see Illman, 1976]

There undoubtedly seems to be an increasing emphasis on coital frequency. People appear to be more and more obsessed by illusory norms. In fact, it is said that doctors and marriage guidance counsellors are worried that envy of the unknown is threatening thousands of insecure marriages (Illman, 1976). There is a preoccupation with performance levels. 'People get the impression from the media that Mrs Average Briton has X number of successful orgasms, and heaven help you if you have more or less.'[3] And this despite the fact that no guidelines for coital frequency can actually be given.[4]

Coupled with this is an expressed concern over coital brevity. For example, extensive research in Italy, fabled for its sensual males, has revealed considerable sexual dissatisfaction. In one survey, 62 per cent of the female respondents reported that intercourse normally lasted no more than two minutes. Some complained that they were treated more like prostitutes. Over half the women interviewed and about a quarter of the men stated that they seldom or never achieved orgasm. In another survey, 19 per cent of the men and 46 per cent of the women said that they faked orgasm, and very similar percentages — 24 and 49 per cent respectively — actually insisted that they usually only made love to keep their partners happy.[5] Male inadequacies are sometimes conveniently attributed to a collocation of religion and maternal indulgence. Women particularly are said to blame a repressive Catholic education and secretive adolescent attitudes towards sex, while the Italian mother is currently held responsible for everything from obesity to impotency.

Again the message is reasonably clear. One would wish to know more about the methodology of the surveys themselves, and 'alien' factors such as the non-response rate which would modify the main conclusions. But, in general, the unease and overall dissatisfaction seem incontrovertible. Problems exist, even among the young, and may be a growing feature of Western society.

There seems to be little doubt that either the problem of sexual unease is more widespread than had been realized or else people are more willing to communicate their anxieties to the appropriate agencies. The Samaritans, who are extremely guarded about their clients, are not infrequently confronted with this type of problem. This has also been the experience of Helpline, the telephone information and counselling service of the Family Planning Association. They have been surprised at the extent of male demand for advice, and report that 75 per cent of their inquiries come from men who are troubled about premature ejaculation and impotence. Helpline's organizer, Mary Capetillo, attributes the problem not so much to speculation about what is going on next door so much as what she terms the 'Robert Redford syndrome', that is to say, husbands failing to match the simulated sexual exploits of their wives' screen heroes.

Indeed, it may be that in films 'the magnificent beast' is taking over from the 'romantic lover'. Actors who used to play the heavy villain now get the hero's part. According to one screen authority, the sexual appetite of men is decreasing and that of the female is dramatically increasing.

> The decline of the male sex drive is now taken so much for granted that the man who *isn't* too tired when he gets home from the office has come to be regarded as some kind of superman . . . [therefore] general female frustration . . . is becoming so widespread [that] sex-starved women fantasise about the gorilla — the primitive brute who will ravish them — rather than the sophisticated and conventionally handsome Prince Charming who will delicately seduce them.[6]

It would appear that this general situation is confirmed by doctors who are actually engaged in the treatment of sexual problems. It is popularly reported that there is 'evidence of general inhibition concerning sex and widespread sexual disability'. Frigidity is said to be the 'commonest disease of women, and impotence afflicts one man in three' (Cauthery, 1975). It is even suggested that the 'copulation explosion' is really something of a myth. The preoccupation with pornography and permissiveness is actually indicative of sexual inadequacy, while orgies and wife-swapping are regarded as frantic attempts at sexual self-treatment. Specialists insist that we are not as sexually sophisticated as we would like to think, and that those who are most at risk are often those who are insecure in other respects. Sexual problems are held to derive from an oppressive sense of competition and may even reflect a general conviction of social and economic failure. More particularly, it may be that many are inhibited by chimerical sexual expectations. They have gradually become fettered by the sexual freedom they are supposed to enjoy.

At a different literary level, there is the esoterica of the 'experience' magazines. These have suddenly proliferated in recent years catering for the verbal titillation of a minority readership. They are entirely concerned with the explicit treatment of sexual themes, and though previously they enjoyed a somewhat subterranean reputation they are now gaining a wider measure of recognition. Their sole *raison d'être* — apart from financial viability — seems to be similar to that of the more commercially oriented soft porn magazines, which, by and large, preach a gospel of hedonistic masculinity. This might be sceptically summarized as the promotion of a 'new' sexual self-awareness which promises personal liberation and self-fulfillment. There may be serious restrictions on individual liberty in the real world where social and economic freedoms are being constantly eroded, but in the private world of the libido true emancipation is possible. However spurious this may sound to those more concerned with political reforms, it does have undeniable compensatory implications. The problem is that the inviolability of this private world is not complete. It is plagued by suspicions and convictions of sexual inadequacy. The pre-conversion life is the sexually unexamined life and is characterized by being experimentally unimaginative and operationally pedestrian. The besetting sin is to be non-orgasmic, so the daimonia of guilt and inhibition must be exorcised by the ritual ministrations of the sexual therapists.

Some writers locate the main area of sexual problems in middle age. They see men in their middle years troubled by depression, doubt and insecurity. What is not clear, however, is whether sexual inadequacy, however defined and empirically established, is the cause or the consequence of what is variously termed the male climacteric, the male menopause or — most vaguely — the mid-life crisis. Professional clinicians are sharply divided on this issue. They tend to agree that there is a disturbing period of change for some men in mid-life, but there is obvious uncertainty as to whether it is due directly to some form of hormonal imbalance. In strictly organic terms, very few men suffer from testicular insufficiency, and even where this does occur it is not possible to connect it specifically with an invariable ageing process.

> As a psychological entity, the male menopause does not exist . . . There are a very small percentage of men, however, between the ages of 55 and 65 who report a sudden reduction of sexual activity associated with mild testicular atrophy. This represents the true male menopause, is organic in origin, and is accompanied by a loss of libido, irritability . . . and impotence.[7]

Others would qualify this and see the male menopause as something that is not simply or even primarily organic but is more a psycho-social condition characterized by anomie and role-uncertainty. The purposeful striving and self-assertion of the early years gradually disappears and is supplanted by the responsiblities and preoccupations of middle age. The confidence of youth gives way to the anxieties of the ageing process (see for example Linacre and Bowskill, 1976).

For women, the cessation of menstruation offers a clear-cut marker of a 'change of life'. For a man there is no specific point or obvious signal, but he may regard his thinning hair and thickening waist as the illest of omens. These augur a crisis of confidence which can manifest itself in sexual terms. Some authorities maintain that sexual self-doubt is possibly the most common symptom of this 'condition'. Men become preoccupied with the question of virility. The possibility — even the actuality — of impotence becomes a matter of primary importance. Dr Herbert Kuperman, a leading New York endocrinologist who specializes in this problem, identifies it as an area of major concern. He estimates that 20 per cent of men between forty-eight and fifty-eight have such a problem, and that this increases to 30—35 per cent between fifty-eight and sixty, and more thereafter (Cooper, 1976). Again, the problem is not primarily attributed to a low level of male hormones, although men do experience an almost imperceptible decline in hormone levels with advancing years. But it is recognized that the matter is far more complex than this. No simple, chemical equation can be applied, especially to the young. All manner of psycho-social factors play a crucial role in the whole process.

There are those who regard the British situation as critical. Dr A.J. Cooper, consultant psychiatrist at Peterborough, estimates that there are 250,000 sexually impotent males in Britain. He attributes this to an amalgam of 'inappropriate sexual education' and the increasing acceptance of a social drug culture, i.e. tranquilizers, alcohol, etc., which deprive the 'male of his masculinity' (Massam, 1972). Again, the claims are sweeping. How is impotency defined? More significantly, how are the figures arrived at? They must be *inferred* from particular clinical case-lists. But over-generalized as these statements are, they do seem to indicate a definite trend.

In all these studies — and certainly in their popular presentation — the interpretations are ambiguous and the diagnoses unclear. This is really all part of the dilemma. What is quite obvious is that problems *do* exist among the young and middle-aged alike, and that they take particular — often sexual — forms. What is not so certain, but what is strongly suggested by the evidence, is that these problems may now be more prevalent than they were. There does not seem to be any really serious doubt about this. A relatively recent investigation conducted by the national magazine *Forum* (see Hodson, 1977) found that half of all male sexual problems presented at clinics concern impotency. The report maintains that more and more men who complain of impotence are under the age of thirty. In fact, when *Forum* asked for 100 volunteers to test a new serum for impotence, 3,457 readers responded, the majority being men under forty. The report further insists that the men who offered themselves for treatment were not just experiencing a 'normal' temporary phase of erectile dysfunction, but were people with a record of repeated failures 'with the regularity of cheap British alarm clocks — unable to go off however carefully you wind them up'. While admitting that there are no precise figures on the actual numbers of impotent men in Britain today, the report refers to the 'alarming new epidemic of impotence in Britain' and rather sensationally concludes that it is 'spreading like the original Black Death' (Hodson, 1977).[8] This view would appear to be confirmed by the experience of Capital Radio in London. When it ran a 'phone-in programme for those with personal, i.e. emotional and sexual, problems and impotence was mentioned, they had 250 letters in the next three days.[9] Similar support comes from another expert, Dr Robert Murphy, an American psychiatrist specializing in sexual problems, who estimates that 'half all males have been impotent at one time or another' and cites the now familiar increasing-female-expectations theory (see Silverberg, 1978).

What is probably more significant is the rise in the number of sex therapy clinics. Sex therapy is now one of our growth industries. Since 1974 it has been partly subsidized by the National Health Service. At that time there were only five state-subsidized clinics; there are now thirty, and by 1980, with a new £30,000 grant, these will probably have increased to forty-two. Supplementarily, there are a number of therapy units attached to the psychiatric departments of many hospitals where sexual problems are regularly treated. In addition to all these public sector operations, there are several private clinics. One of the best known, that of Dr Patricia Gillan in Harley Street, has been reported as having a two-month waiting list. The Institute of Sex Research and Education at Birmingham is in a similar position. Dr Martin Cole, a lecturer in biology at the University of Aston, who runs the Institute, concentrates mainly on male sexual dysfunction. He has a list of some 2,000 men, of whom only about a quarter have had treatment so far.[10] The problem here is clearly one of time and the availability of suitable therapists.

Whether the incidence of impotence assumes the magnitude that some writers adduce is debatable. An inference from particular cases is not a random survey, and numerical speculations are not carefully calculated statistics. Indeed, the very nature of the phenomenon precludes these possibilities. But the wealth of evidence is there. The inquiries in newspapers and magazines,[11] the growing numbers presenting themselves for treatment — all indicate an alarmingly familiar and growing trend. That a problem exists is no longer in dispute, but the actual *extent* of the problem is unknown and almost certainly unknowable. The point that is really in contention is why the problem should exist at all. How can we account for it? What theories are held to 'explain' it? And can these in any way be related to significant changes that are taking place in modern society?

5. Case Histories

The problem of male impotence, particularly erectile dysfunction, is receiving increasing attention by doctors and psychiatrists whose work is clinically based. Their findings are not derived from the kind of survey samples from which it is normally possible to extrapolate trends for a larger population. Indeed, in this area it can even prove rather fruitless to advertise for respondents; impotent males are hardly likely to declare their failures any more than premature ejaculators are to confess their shortcomings. Other than the postal survey technique (for example the *Forum* survey — see Hodson, 1977), which must have a limited usefulness, researchers have to be content with self-selected samples of presenting patients. And these almost certainly represent a mere fraction of the total dysfunctional population.

Those who actively seek treatment may well include those of the auto-voyeuristic fringe who gain a certain mental gratification from detailing their sexual non-experiences, a form of quiet exhibitionism which has its own sexual rewards. Some others may have volunteered for therapy because of the intriguing prospect of visual aid and surrogate treatment — although these may be very much a minority. In short, much of the research being currently conducted is arguably based on unrepresentative groups, and its findings will necessarily be coloured by the 'confined' nature of the information that is given. These limitations are reduced where partners are involved, or where surrogates can be trusted for reliable reports, but even in these cases it is impossible to eliminate entirely the possibility of bias. As we shall see, the whole business of analysis is a highly subjective operation.

It is for this reason that this discussion would not be complete without some case histories. These are profiles of men in quite different circumstances who have all experienced, or are experiencing, their own forms of sexual dysfunction. In some instances it might be more accurate to say that they are experiencing similar erectile difficulties, which are symptomatic of different basic problems. They have been chosen quite arbitrarily, but they do represent different age categories and their circumstances are very dissimilar.[1] What their stories exemplify is the fact that there is no 'type' of male who is singular or stereotypical, or who is completely immune from the condition. All men are potential victims, but, by the same token, most men who are victims are potentially curable. It may be that the cause of the problem in the majority of cases is 'purely' psychological, although some authorities disagree with this; for example, Martin Cole, who runs the Institute for Sex Research and Education, believes that eventually we may find that as many as one-third of all cases are attributable to some kind of hormonal disturbance or deficiency. But as yet this is a minority view. This study wishes to stress psycho-social factors, and is primarily concerned with the *context* in which the phenomenon occurs and the *forms* in which it is expressed.

It would perhaps be as well, therefore, to look at some instances of 'straight' impotence first, those cases in which we are dealing with unambiguous erectile problems.

CASE B: The Ageing Male

The subject at the time of interview was a retired policeman of seventy-two. He was married, and his wife was still living; there had been just one child who had died when only five years of age. Since that time their intercourse had been conducted without the use of contraceptives. In his army service during the war the husband had some casual sexual experiences, possibly with prostitutes — this was not made exactly clear. Other than this there was no admission of any extra-marital affairs.

Until the onset of his sexual difficulties intercourse had taken place about once a fortnight. But even in these early years of the marriage there had been a marked tendency towards premature ejaculation. His wife had apparently been uncomplaining about this, and the question of her own sexual satisfaction was never discussed. He is not even sure when or whether she ever achieved orgasm. It appears to have been something that they both found difficult to recognize. Possibly it was not so much a matter of lack of concern on his part, as an unwillingness to face the issues involved. A guarded sexual reticence seems to have been part of their normal routine. Self-examination would not have been considered necessary or even proper in the circumstances.

At the age of forty-six the subject was found to have syphilis, possibly as the result of his earlier sexual encounters. This was treated medically with apparent success, but there is little doubt that this condition gave an added element of uncertainty to marital relations. About six years after this he developed a nervous condition which never seems to have been successfully diagnosed. Obviously, the possibility of an ominous connection between this and the previous venereal infection cannot be completely ruled out. For this nervous disability drugs were prescribed, and by the time of the interview the subject had been taking pheno-barbitone for about twenty years.

Erectile problems began quite suddenly when he was

fifty-nine. Unlike some cases of impotence, especially in ageing males, there was no gradual onset of the condition. Normal sexual relations were not punctuated by occasional failures. For no apparent reason, erection suddenly became difficult. There was still a certain amount of love-play, but actual intercourse was out of the question. Masturbation sometimes produced a partial erection and now and then ejaculation occurred. Again, his wife was understanding and never reproached him. There seemed to be no reason to consult anyone about it, not even a doctor. He did not seem particularly distressed about it and simply ascribed it to old age. The situation was seen as unfortunate but 'natural', and left at that.

The physical and chemical changes that accompany the ageing process would seem to be an obvious answer in this case, although the fact that there was sudden erectile failure which then persisted perhaps indicates rather more than this. After the interview an appointment was made for the subject to discuss his problem with a doctor. She too advanced the ageing hypothesis and maintained that it was not at all abnormal for a man to have this problem in his late fifties. It was also discovered that, when he was sixty-eight, he had had an operation for an enlarged prostate gland, and almost any operative interference in this region with the sympathetic nerve supply would probably make erection impossible. He was not told this at the time of the operation, probably on the assumption that it did not really matter too much at that age, and that as the patient already had a history of impotence he was not actually going to lose anyway.

These physical factors were obviously the cause of the problem at the time of the interview, but it is worth noting that the problem had existed for some nine years prior to the operation. The doctor confirmed that during this time the patient's condition was almost certainly aggravated by many years of barbiturate medication, a contingency about which he had no knowledge and about which he had never been warned.

As we have already seen, erectile dysfunction is not a necessary or inevitable concomitant of old age, but the incidence is significantly greater at this time. This is due partly to the hormonal changes that accompany the ageing process, and not infrequently to the presence of other physical problems that are more prevalent in later years. But what should not be overlooked are the psychological implications. Ageing men are all too conscious of their own physical deterioration. They are well aware that they are no longer so appealing to prospective partners. Though old themselves, they can still find the young attractive; though not particularly desirable themselves, they can still desire — and this desire may not extend to their legitimate or available partners, who are presumably ageing too. In short, their impotence, at least in part, may be a function of insufficient or inappropriate stimulation. Normally, a condition of erectile adequacy is strong sexual excitement. But how is this possible without a suitable object of desire? Masters and Johnson note that this may be a key factor with some older men; they will perform better with younger partners. It is certainly no accident that in social circumstances where men are rich or powerful enough to take younger wives and mistresses they often do so. But this is not normally so easy in our kind of society. So what is left for the older man? He can always resort to the Ladies Directory or the sauna, or treat himself to lonely masturbatory consolations. Failing this, he must — sadly — be content with the purely vicarious experiences of the media, or recourse to the solace of recollection.

CASE C: The Widowed Male

This man was a moulder by trade, but had been in the

army for most of his working life. Though only fifty-six at the time of the interview, he was now effectively retired owing to ill health. He was drawing an army pension, and was becoming anxious about money, estimating that after paying his mortgage he had only about £16 a week left to cover all his expenses. His wife had died about five years previously, and he was now living alone in a small suburban house. There had been two daughters of the marriage, both of whom had now married themselves. The younger daughter had only recently left home, and visited her father quite frequently, but the elder daughter had been diagnosed as schizophrenic and was undergoing treatment.

During his service in the army he had prided himself on his prowess with women. 'I was a good lover — I liked to take an hour over it — but I enjoyed the chase more than the actual performance.' In these years there had been occasional instances of erectile difficulty. He recalled a particular experience in 1964 in a Malaysian brothel when he felt extremely distressed because he could only 'manage' a partial erection. He was further humiliated by the attitude of the girls, who appeared to have no sympathy with his condition. On these excursions he often drank fairly heavily, and he admits that in such situations he tended to use drink 'as an alibi' for his failure. He appreciates now that alcohol may have been only a contributory factor, but at the time it seems to have provided a convenient excuse, although even then there were vestigial doubts.

In 1969, he left the army and became a stores supervisor for a transport authority. At about the same time, he experienced renewed sexual problems. Erectile difficulties became more frequent. His wife was very understanding, and they both attributed his problem to the stress and uncertainty of leaving the Forces and trying to settle into a new job. It was regarded as a transitional phase which would pass. He and his wife had always enjoyed good sexual relations until this time, but that was when he was on leave, and this gave a special piquance to their lovemaking. When he was home *all* the time, and sex was no longer rationed, he found this kind of routinized domesticity an unfamiliar experience.

In 1972 his wife died after a lengthy illness. Despite his pecadillos with other women he appears to have had a genuine affection for her, and he obviously missed her a great deal. After a period of unhappiness and indecision, he began to frequent local night-clubs openly looking for women. His feeling of loneliness led him to join an Introductions Club, and in 1974 he met a woman whom he 'courted for nine months'. She was just a little younger than he, fifty-two and was separated from her husband. He again had erectile difficulties, and again drink may have played some part in his failure. It is quite apparent that they went drinking together, and he insists that he was often put off by her manner, especially when she was drunk. She, for her part, was distressed by the ultimately unsatisfactory nature of their relationship.

By this time he had left his job and tried to run a small business of his own supplying stretch covers, but it was not a success, and he soon found himself in debt. Needless to say, these business worries did nothing to help his domestic—sexual situation. He eventually decided to consult a doctor, but was simply told not to worry and that the condition would correct itself.

In 1975, possibly because it seemed lucrative but mainly because it offered a complete change, he took a job in Iran. There he became very fond of a Persian woman, and he brought both her and her daughter back to live with him in England. Again, despite both attraction and affection, he still had sexual problems, and finally she returned in despair to Iran. Since that time there had been other women, some of whom he had simply picked up in public houses: in 1976 a forty-eight year-old divorcee and, more recently, yet another woman who also appears to have been a near-alcoholic. Often the women in question were willing enough sexually, and sometimes they were actively enthusiastic. On rare occasions he had effective erections and consequent masturbation, but since the death of his wife he had never had successful intercourse with anyone.

In 1976 also, he had a heart attack and was compelled to retire from work. He was still able to go out from time to time and still enjoyed the company of women, but had now become virtually resigned to his condition.

It would be tempting to see this case in terms of repressed guilt. Here is a man who had spent the greater part of his married life away from home. He had not given his wife and family the attention they needed and perhaps deserved. Now both daughters had left home, one was undergoing treatment for a condition which, he may feel, might not have developed with more balanced parental care. What was worse, his wife had died. He had not treated her particularly well; instead of settling down with her and the children after the war he had rejoined the army. Again, she was left with the main responsibility for rearing the family while he enjoyed the qualified freedoms of the professional soldier. More specifically, he had often been unfaithful with other women, and not infrequently they were little more than prostitutes who did not compare with his wife in strictly qualitative terms. Now she was dead. She had never had much of a life, but it was now no longer possible to make it up to her — or to the children, for that matter.

As a widower, he became lonely and depressed. Yet he couldn't be expected to remain celibate for the rest of his life, so he went out to clubs and pubs, and joined a friendship group hoping to make the right kind of contacts. But the sexual prospects were limited. He was now an ageing male, so the field was becoming more restricted. He was no longer sexually confident, but he was sure of his ability to chat-up the available talent. As failure followed failure, it is quite possible that the need to 'cure' his problem became as important as the need for companionship. He thought it might be all right if he found the right woman, but with few exceptions the women he encountered were, in their own ways, as pathetic as himself.

This kind of explanation seems superficial and a little simplistic, but it is persuasive in the absence of anything better. It does not fit with all the facts. There is evidence of erectile dysfunction in earlier years, and certainly during later married life. Given that there had been a medical consultation — although apparently no actual *examination* — it can perhaps be assumed that there was no direct organic reason for impotence. On the other hand, alcohol probably played a part, but this may only have been a contributory factor, which could be made to bear as much of the blame as the occasion required.

What we have here then is the case of a man who genuinely cared for his wife whom he regarded as a loyal partner and a good woman. But she was not enough. She was not particularly exciting sexually — at least, not for *him*. He had not wanted to be bound to the home or to a single sexual outlet. But now he had problems, now he was alone, and now he had regrets which affected every subsequent performance.

In a sense, this is not really an explanation, merely an approach to an understanding. It is natural for the subject to think that it might all have been different had his wife not died. She was a sympathetic person and perhaps they could have solved their problems together. Perhaps. It is so easy to rewrite history. Any objective reconstruction would not necessarily encourage such optimism. The sexual urgency may never be rekindled once the excitement has gone.

CASE D: The Womanizing Male

In this case we have a mature student, who in his middle twenties quite unexpectedly found himself confronted with the problem of erectile dysfunction. His general background is unexceptional, but the events immediately preceding and accompanying his first 'failure' are perhaps significant.

The subject had already been divorced for about two years when he commenced his studies. His marriage, which had also lasted about two years, he now regarded as well and truly finished. In his pre-college days he had been self-employed, and his various small entrepreneurial activities had even extended to wholesaling pornographic literature. He had grown tired of this kind of life and had begun to aspire to some form of social work, for which he needed the necessary formal qualifications. At the time of the interview he had been a student for several months, and was finding some difficulty in settling down in an unfamiliar environment with even more unfamiliar subjects. The discipline of study was new, and he was very aware of the paradoxical nature of his own situation; he was more mature and worldly-wise than the majority of his fellow students, yet his relative lack of formal education made him feel rather inferior in an academic community.

By his own account, he had had considerable sexual experience. This had begun well before he was married, and his catholic sexual attitudes may have contributed in part to the break-up of the marriage. Until the onset of erectile difficulties, his promiscuous approach to sexual relations had continued unabated. He had established an on-going relationship with a married woman besides maintaining his retinue of casual acquaintances. A familiar feature of his repertoire was to pick up likely talent at a dance, and complete the evening with a more-or-less successful seduction. It was during one of these opportunistic encounters that his problems first began.

The particularly interesting thing is that his first experience of erectile dysfunction happened suddenly and unexpectedly. As far as one can ascertain, it was quite foreign to his normal pattern of operation. It took place about a year after the break-up of his marriage, when he was driving a casual acquaintance home from a dance. He had been drinking, but not to excess. It was a long drive, and he was tired — all factors that can militate against sexual success. On the other hand, this was going to be no fumbling operation in the back of a car. He had his own house, he had seclusion — conditions that he regarded as 'ideal'. The lady in question was attractive and sexually experienced, although she did insist on talking about a relationship with another man with whom she was not particularly happy. In the preliminaries immediately prior to intercourse there was no erectile response. No sheath was being used — a factor that can lead to hesitation and uncertainty for some couples. Both attempted to remedy the situation by pausing and then applying the customary stimulatory techniques — but without success. The girl seemed very sympathetic, and did her best to make him feel that it was just one of those unfortunate one-off occasions. But it wasn't. Not long afterwards they repeated their attempts — this time in a car — but again without success. He had hoped this would rectify matters, and this time there was a partial erection, but not sufficient for intromission. The girl remained understanding, but this did little to assuage his humiliation or lessen his uncomprehending sense of failure.

For about a month he had no success with any *other* girls. Thereafter, for no accountable reason, all went well with some girls and not with others. His second complete failure happened about two months after the first. Again, it took place at his house, but with a different girl, who also had another steady boyfriend. She too was sexually experienced and sympathetic to his problem. The third complete failure took place in his car with yet another girl whom he described as 'easy'. There was no hostility or ridicule, but she was not as understanding as his previous partners.

He was determined to conquer the problem and, in effect, tested himself in as wide a series of circumstances as he could. His erectile responses became quite unpredictable. He had various failures, partial failures and complete non-response in both coital and non-coital situations with a number of different partners. But during this whole period, which lasted about twelve months, he carried on a regular affair with his married girlfriend without any acknowledged problems whatsoever. He made no excuses to himself for his condition, and with gradual perseverence seemed to overcome his difficulties. But the case has an interesting postscript. Having been virtually free from trouble for a year or so before interview, he found some return of the problem after having discussed it in detail. This was only temporary, but it shows that, contrary to the views of some analysts, recollection may not be cathartic but may be actually reinforcing in its effects.

Yet again, in this case no obvious explanation presents itself. Perhaps there was, in fact, no *one* cause, but a complex of causes. The circumstances in which intercourse was attempted were, in most cases, conducive to successful sex. Privacy, comfort and little fear of interruption should have added to the occasion. (Of course, there are some people who perversely relish the prospect of sex in difficult circumstances because it adds a kind of exquisite tension to their activities, but this does not seem to have been the case here.)

Some might argue that for a once-married man to bring girls to his own house is to court trouble by association. Again, the inhibiting-sense-of-guilt argument has a certain cogency, either in relation to his ex-wife or his regular girlfriend, who had also used the house. Indeed, the fact that he was able to continue this reasonably stable sexual relationship without problems suggests that this argument has some validity, but nothing conclusive can be determined.

Some theorists insist that womanizing tendencies are really a canalization of deep-seated potency fears (see Main, 1976, pp. 104ff.). This Don Juan complex actually cloaks a gnawing conviction that one day the system might fail, so moving from girl to girl is simply one way of proving oneself to oneself, or, on another analysis, of maintaining a kind of coital death-wish. There may be more than a germ of truth in this approach; certainly, fear of failure appears to be a significant feature of some male sexual activity. But for the theorists, it's a fail-safe model. If you don't womanize you either lack libido or are afraid to try your luck; if you do womanize you are just manifesting a basic sexual insecurity. And this is not to mention the fact that, on either reading, you could be a latent homosexual! Either way, you just can't win. The Don Juan theory[2] has interesting possibilities, but little more than this. If a man is super-active sexually, whatever other problems he may have, he certainly does not suffer from erectile dysfunction.

It would seem too that in this case partner response was not an important factor. Generally speaking, the women in question were helpful and sympathetic, and used their experience to try to restore his apparently waning sexual capacities. We have to say 'apparently', because we are not really sure just what his problem was on any one occasion. Certainly his erectile difficulties were irrefutable, but why did he 'go off the boil' at the crucial moment? It may initially have been something as simple as physical over-indulgence. He was already maintaining a regular sexual relationship; perhaps he just over-reached himself on a particular occasion, and had trouble thereafter. It need require only one instance to establish a failure syndrome where the effect becomes the cause of future dysfunction. And this may hit the super-active male that much harder simply because it is unexpected and is alien to all his previous experience.

It might now be instructive to look at the 'grey areas' of sexual dysfunction; those cases that are perhaps not technically classifiable as impotence, but are nevertheless germaine to our discussion. We have already seen that there are instances — as in cases of paraphilia — in which operational 'abnormality' may be a symptom of underlying sexual difficulties.[3] These sexual variations, or what might be seen as deviations, may not be thought of as impotence, as strictly defined; but they do have related implications.

CASE E: The Virgin Male

In a technical sense, this is not a straightforward case of sexual impotence. It is not a problem of erectile dysfunction, as such, but the case of a person with the apparent psychological inability to form those relationships that necessarily precede sexual contacts. Sometimes the term 'heterophobic' (literally, a fear of the other kind) is used to denote those individuals who cannot bring themselves to a pre-sexual situation with partners to whom they are often mentally attracted. These are often males who frequently *want* to make such contacts. They may even fantasize and imagine themselves in sexual situations — often for masturbatory purposes. But they cannot, for undetermined reasons, actualize their wishes.

At the time of interview, the subject was a twenty-three-year-old trainee teacher. He was a well qualified physics graduate who had been finding teaching practice hard going at a local secondary school, and was beginning to wonder about his general suitability for the job. This is not an uncommon reaction to teaching practices; having emerged from academic incubation, aspirants usually find their ideas and their ideals challenged at this point, but in this case the uncertainty seemed particularly marked.

He was born into a practising Catholic family. His parents had married comparatively late, and he was their only child. The father was a teacher himself who was now nearing retirement age. (The subject seemed to think it significant to mention that his father's sister was a deaf mute who lived in a mental hospital — perhaps to indicate that there were other 'abnormalities' in the family). He regarded his father as 'educated' and tolerant, and generally enjoyed good relations with him. Towards his mother he was much more ambivalent. He described her as neurotic and working-class, someone he respected as a mother, but not as a person. She had uninformed 'Puritan attitudes', which she would announce but rarely discuss. Disputes took place, but the mother seemed incapable of rational argument. And the situation was aggravated by her extreme possessiveness, which he bitterly resented. There were no arguments with his father, who — he insisted — took a humanistic and intelligent approach, especially in matters of religion and morality.

In his formative years he was very influenced by what he understood as Catholic teaching. Sex was a questionable area, and sexual contacts outside the sacrament of marriage were wrong. He had never had any direct sexual instruction, but remembered reading a passage about sex in a book when he was about eight years old, which shocked him deeply.

As he matured, his attitudes towards sex became

completely ambivalent. He claims to have been attracted to girls from the age of seven, and continues to feel ashamed that he wants them. In his early years he had some homosexual experiences, and was quite capable of erections in these circumstances. On one occasion he was seduced by an older boy, and they indulged in masturbation and fellatio but not buggery. From this period onwards there has been no overt homosexuality; indeed, he insists that there has been no desire for such relationships.

Living at home again, his parents never openly questioned his apparent lack of interest in girls, and certainly never encouraged him to bring any to the house. Recently he has become involved with an amateur dramatic group, which gives him ample scope with the opposite sex. These play rehearsals do give an opportunity for mild sexual contact and, in effect, legitimate certain preliminary sexual activities. But he finds simulation of this kind something of an 'effort'. It does not excite him, and does not produce erections; it merely gives rise to secret fantasies, which then just 'fade away'.

He never reads pornography, but occasionally has 'wet dreams'. He can get sexually excited, and sometimes masturbates, but this does not lead to orgasm. There has been no medical consultation about this, and he is careful not to confide his fears to others.

The subject is aware of the paradoxes of his own situation. He remains intrigued by the sexual possibilities that are open to him, but is still proud of his own chastity. He has developed an interest in the psychology of men—women relationships, especially since being at university, yet still holds himself aloof from any personal involvement. He would like a relationship, but is not sure whether it would be, could be, or even *should* be a sexual relationship. Sex fascinates him, yet it is somehow beneath him. His superior view of its 'sordidness' gives him a false sense of invulnerability.

Here again, the lines of explanation may seem to be fairly obvious. But there are, in fact, several choices. No *one* clear pattern can actually be discerned. The least likely is that there is a physical — possibly hormonal — deficiency of some kind. The subject has not sought the help of a doctor, so it can be naturally assumed that there has been no medical examination. The matter of possible organic dysfunction must therefore remain an open question. But in the light of more plausible alternative explanations, this must be a doubtful starter.

Some suitably adapted variant of the oedipal complex might prove to be a more likely prospect. Certainly the Freudian psychotherapists would probably opt for this approach. The ambivalent attitudes of the subject to his mother, their love—hate relationship — all would fit the pattern. The subject's inability to form satisfactory relationships with girls, his lack of 'normal' excitation in drama group-simulated situations, appear to point to the well known mother-comparison problems. There are, of course, the complications of his apparent latent homosexuality, but these too can be conveniently accommodated within the same general theoretical model. Psychoanalysis has it all ways, but its conclusions are entirely hypothetical. The oedipal wish — the suggested desire of a boy for his mother — is simply an explanatory construct with unproven universal applications. It is only necessary to reiterate that, as a key to understanding particular cases, it can never be empirically validated, and that as a general theory it can be no more than an intellectualized hunch.

A more sociological approach would tend to concentrate on the subject's upbringing, particularly on the role of religion as an agency of socialization. The inability of the subject to resolve the conflicting norms of society and the Church may not fully explain his sexual problems, but they do suggest the general direction in which an explanation might be sought.

The next two case histories are based upon interviews with wives only. This gives the cases an interesting slant even if many of the important facts remain unknown.

CASE F: The Habituated Male

This subject is extremely difficult to assess. He is forty-three and a sales assistant with a nationalized company. He has been married for nineteen years to a woman just one year younger than himself, and they have a daughter now in her teens.

It is reasonably clear that the subject had an 'unhappy childhood'. He came from a broken home and had rather poor relations with his mother. He had 'only an elementary education' and — according to his wife — this is a source of some regret to him, especially when he compares his own achievement and job potential with hers. Much of his time is now taken up with a variety of social and recreational activities. He takes his wife to occasional parties, and they like to 'go out for a drink', although he does not appear to drink to excess. His absorbing outside interests have recently centred on darts, sailing and work with Round Table.

The nature and extent of his pre-marital sexual experience is not known. It is possible that his first 'real experiences' were with his wife before marriage; she certainly gives the impression that she organized his sex life in those days. This seems a little odd because, on her own admission, it was often spontaneous and had the high-risk element of not involving the use of contraceptives.

Nowadays sex is still spontaneous but is less frequent. There is little or no preliminary fore-play, no 'touching below the waist' — not even kissing. Furthermore, there is no 'profession of love', which the wife obviously expects to sanctify the occasion. In short, sexual activity has become perfunctory and 'remote'. The husband has some erectile difficulties when he tries to accommodate his wife against his own inclinations, but his main problem is in achieving orgasm. His wife's orgasm is usually brought about manually or in the woman superior position, which normally allows her more control of movement and gives extra clitoral stimulation. Apparently, the husband does not request or require sexual aids of any kind, and certainly no pornographic materials are involved, although he does often like to use mirrors. A further point of interest here is that he does seem to respond more readily to the prospect of sex in semi-public situations, say in a field. The possibility of detection appears to add spice to the occasion. The idea of being seen or, conversely, of 'seeing' oneself — as with the mirrors — is obviously a source of added excitement.

The wife considers herself a reasonably highly sexed person, and despairs of her husband's seeming indifference. She obviously regards her husband as rather uneducated sexually, and professes that she only discovered the pleasures of oral sex a few years ago with another man. She reads soft porn, mainly *Playgirl,* which readily displays male genitalia. She masturbates frequently, and over the last five years or so has had irregular extra-marital affairs. She is involved professionally with health and sex education, which might be regarded as one form of canalization for her interests. In fact, her extra-marital encounters usually take place at conferences that she attends in connection with her work. It is fairly clear that she looks forward to these occasions, and although she does not regard herself as being in any way promiscuous, she sometimes arranges things so that the possibility of extracurricular activity with a known partner becomes a virtual certainty.

In this case, there do not seem to be any of the obvious physical complications. He drinks 'regularly', but apparently within the bounds of moderation. His wife's health too is good; she is a little overweight and has had thrush briefly, but not enough to impair normal sexual relations. The husband has had a vasectomy, but there is no evidence that this has had any deleterious psychological effects, and he does not regard this as in any way detracting from his manliness. Indeed, the fact that mechanical methods of contraception are now no longer necessary should enhance the sexual possibilities and facilitate his slightly eccentric sense of spontaneity.

His attitude to his wife's sexual proclivities is uncertain. He is somewhat cool, almost impervious to her advances, and gives the impression of lacking sexual drive. He knows that his wife 'pets' at parties that they both attend, but 'he just does not seem to mind'. On the other hand, he does not appear to be aware of any actual infidelity — however that is to be defined — although he obviously suspects it. He says that, *if* it happens, he just does not want to know. But the question is: does he really want it to happen? And if he thought it did would it afford him some inner, vicarious, pleasure? Or is the explanation much more prosaic, namely that normal marital relations are simply wearing thin, and he is actually becoming indifferent to his wife's sexual desires, however directed? It is not unusual for years of habituation to generate some kind of reaction eventually. Interest is probably beginning to wane, and he may secretly welcome the possibility of his wife's unfaithfulness because it gives him an 'out' from the ongoing tedium of predictable marital sex.

In qualification of this view, it must be noted that he does not appear to have been involved in any extra-marital affairs himself. Nor does he seem to be seeking any alternative outlet other than his preoccupying leisure activities. Perhaps these are a form of sublimation; perhaps they are an escape from the otherwise intolerable suspicion of his own inadequacy. On this point, it must be stressed that his perceptions of himself and his own life-style are important, and — as far as can be assessed — he does not regard himself as being at all abnormal sexually. He does not bemoan his fate or regard himself as having a 'condition'. Possibly, like many men, he takes the view that this is the way things are at *that* age when you have been married *that* long.

Case G: The Indifferent Husband

The situation reported here is now *passé*. This is a brief account of a wife's experience with her first husband, and the incidents concerned are now several years old. Nevertheless, it is instructive as another variation on the dysfunction theme.

Except that he had a rather dominating mother, the male in question seems to have had an unremarkable upbringing. He is said to be attractive to women and to have had several affairs before marrying the interviewee when he was twenty-three and she was eighteen. When they had met she was still a virgin, and prior to marriage they had lived together for three months, during which time there had been no sexual problems. Indeed, she insists that things started to go wrong only once they were married.

During their married life, there had never been any obvious erectile difficulties. Again, the problem seems to have been a general lack of libido. Intervals between actual coitus lengthened until they reached five to six months. These were not punctuated by any physical alternatives such as oral sex; the only occasional substitute was auto-masturbation for the male. And in the very rare circumstances when the wife took the initiative, her advances were repulsed. There was no known paraphilia of a deviant or variant nature. Certainly no visual aids were ever used. When intercourse did occur no contraceptive methods of any kind were employed.

For some time, the husband refused to talk about the matter, and it began to sour the entire relationship. When the wife complained, he actually suggested that she should consider having an affair with someone. After a decent interval she decided to take him at his word. Eventually, while still married, she had a baby by the man who is now her second husband. Later on, within the same period, the husband began living with another girl, but the wife thinks that he was probably not sleeping with her as she was still technically a minor. Other than this instance, there is no reason to suppose that the husband was ever unfaithful during their three years of marriage.

Until the wife actually sought sexual consolation elsewhere, she believes that her husband — 'in a strange kind of way' — really did want to make the marriage work despite his manifest lack of sexual interest. She explains this by assuming that his problem was specifically sexual; that he was, in fact, suffering from some form of impotency, and that he made few sexual overtures because he was afraid of failure. Why this should be so is uncertain. She insists that there was no drink problem, but recalls that at about the same time that the difficulties first became apparent her husband was especially anxious about settling in at a new job. It is conceivable, of course, that an initial failure at this time might have precipitated a syndrome of anticipated failure as time went on, but there is no specific evidence to support this.

The cynical adage that relationships based on love are ruined by marriage obviously contains a germinal truth. It certainly seems to be pertinent to this particular case. Until marriage, the husband enjoyed good sexual relations not only with his wife-to-be but also with an assortment of other women. After marriage, his need for yet further variety may have precipitated what she interpreted as a 'problem'. Even his altruistic — or perhaps astute — suggestion that his wife should take a lover has a self-justifying potential. It also has paraphilic overtones. The wife recollected how stimulated he was when she revealed something of her own extra-marital sexual excursions.

After the split in their relationship, the husband was more willing to discuss the problem with her. He explained it in terms of 'feeling threatened' by her expanding sexual experience. Be that as it may, she insists that he certainly could not have felt threatened by her increasing sexual *demands,* as she was very reluctant to make any positive advances in the circumstances.

Perhaps the truth in this case is that there was really no problem at all. Or, to put it more precisely, that the problem was in the marriage, not in any specific sexual dysfunctionality. The wife is obviously reluctant to see it in these terms, but it will certainly bear this kind of interpretation. It may be that what the wife regarded as her husband's 'difficulties' were really his way of extricating himself from a difficult situation. What had originally been a marital misjudgement had eventually become an ongoing predicament — there was no way of effectively divorcing the sexual issues from the domestic ones.

The cases we have considered represent a spectrum of dysfunctional possibilities. They have ranged from 'straight' erectile problems probably associated with age and excessive use of commonly prescribed drugs to the uncertainties of inappropriate socialization and inadequate sex drive. The purely physical elements — the ageing process, hormonal imbalance, the effects of drugs or alcohol — are difficult to assess, and are almost certainly not the main problem of most men. What is much more pertinent is the context in which their sexuality is expressed. When we refer, for instance, to a man as having a low sex drive, what are we really saying? Are we saying any more than that for certain — possibly identifiable — reasons he is not sexually aroused? We must always bear in mind that there may be physiological implications, but we must not discount the possibility of psycho-social factors. These are not simply residual considerations; they may well be crucial to a true understanding of the situation.

If there is one point that emerges time and time again in the investigation of male sexual dysfunction, it is the necessity of adequate and appropriate stimuli. For most men this presumably means having a suitable partner. But this, in turn, may also imply having either a change of partner or even a variety of partners. There are, of course, instances where fear of failure actually produces failure, even when the partner is eminently suitable. It is here that therapy can play a part. There are a number of strategies that can be employed in these and similar circumstances with varying degrees of success. But before we consider these, it might be instructive to look at some of the theories that have been offered to explain the phenomenon itself.

6. Theories of Male Sexual Dysfunction

Science abhors a cognitive vacuum, and no more so than in the study of aberrant sexual behaviour. Understandings and misunderstandings proliferate. So where no single satisfactory explanation exists, several have to do.

In studies of impotence, the whole business is both simplified and complicated by the work of professional practitioners: simplified because the possible therapies are conveniently reduced to variants of a few standardized approaches, and complicated because these do not necessarily increase our real understanding of the underlying conditions. The basic purpose of therapy is to improve performance, so techniques are carefully designed to engender or restore a sense of sexual confidence. As we shall see, a reassuring number of patients do respond effectively to behavioural and other treatments. But the reasons for any particular individual's original loss of confidence may never actually be discovered. The physical condition may tell us nothing about its genesis. The effects can often be successfully treated, but the contributory causes may never be fully known. It therefore remains forever uncertain whether or not the same hidden anxieties will one day reassert themselves. In a curious way, the effect can become the cause.

One further preliminary point should be made. What are we actually doing when we advance theories about *any*thing? In brief, a theory may be regarded as a formal explanatory proposition based upon known principles. To this extent, it is much less tentative than a hypothesis, which is really an unsupported theory, and merely constitutes the starting point of an investigation. It is important first of all that a theory should be falsifiable (cf. the work of Sir Karl Popper, particularly Popper, 1968). A statement can be regarded as 'scientific' only when it is open to validation or invalidation — and certainly to modification — on experimental grounds. Statements that seem to be commonsensically or even consensually 'true', such as 'Beethoven is a good composer' or 'stealing is wrong', are not capable of falsification and are not therefore scientifically valid. Ethical and aesthetic statements naturally fall into this category, although these may involve kinds of truth that are not susceptible to scientific methods of investigation (see Carlton, 1973). Similarly, statements that seem patently false, such as 'I receive telepathic instructions from extra-terrestial beings', can never be conclusively proved or disproved because, in the nature of the case, the claim in question is not amenable to experimental verification.

It is not uncommon in the study of sexual behaviour to find numerous statements that are quite unscientific in this sense. This is particularly so in the case of causal explanations. For instance, the much-vaunted relationship between inadequate sexual performance and childhood guilt is notoriously difficult to establish. How can there ever be any more than a *plausible* connection between, say, a nagging adolescent conscience about masturbation and the inability to control ejaculation in the middle years? Pseudo-psychological theorizing of this kind is really part of an ideological backlash from those who regard the 'new sexuality' as an implicit critique of religious ideas (see for instance Simmons, 1970). Doesn't everybody know that nuns take long and vigorous walks simply to sublimate their resurgent sexual instincts? This sort of thing is superficially persuasive, but is really just one more instance of the isigetical tendency to 'see' causal connections where they do not necessarily exist. Such relationships are quite incapable of demonstration. Perhaps it is remotely conceivable that every all-in wrestler is really a latent homosexual, but a suspicion is hardly an explanation.

In advancing some theories of impotence, we are not simply classifying *types* of impotence.[1] Theories are, at best, very tentative affairs, and certainly there is no *one* unifying theory of impotence that can be advanced to cover every experiential contingency. In this part of the discussion, then, we will be thinking only incidentally of types of impotence. What will concern us specifically will be the *types of theories* that are held to account for it. Typologies of this kind can be very useful in that they help us to order our thinking about the phenomenon in question. Their clarificatory function is to prepare the way for more detailed investigation. Indeed, there are those who insist that the classification of objects involves an implicit prediction of how they will behave in given circumstances. And this may be analagous to the classification of situations (see de Jouvenel, 1963, p. 63). Typologies, therefore, are not mere inventions, but are ways of reducing complex and often conflicting data to manageable proportions. But it should be reiterated that not one of the theories of causation that we are about to consider can be regarded as wholly adequate *in itself,* and that even taken together they can do little more than act as preliminary pointers to further study.

PHYSIOLOGICAL THEORIES

These have already been quite fully treated in earlier sections of our discussion. The term 'physiological' is used here in contra-distinction to complementary theories, which tend to emphasize the interplay of socio-psychological variables in the occurance of impotence.

The physiological category includes such factors as the ageing process, organic disease, and the often necessary administration of drugs. In relatively rare circumstances it may also be concerned with hormonal imbalance and physical deformity or deficiency. It also covers the abuse of various so-called stimulants such as tobacco, alcohol and cannabis. For example, it is reported that research carried out in the United States in February 1976 showed that alcohol is responsible for destroying by a factor of five the amount of male sex hormone, testosterone, with consequent effects on potency (Hodson, 1977). Similarly, it was found that after nine weeks cannabis reduced testosterone levels by a third when smoked regularly by male researchers.

This category must also include, by definition, the effects of exposure to many of the drugs and compounds used in modern industry. For instance, a case was reported in 1970 of seven men in Scotland who became impotent after handling styrene (Hodson, 1977). Similar concern has been expressed about chemicals currently in use in agriculture, and it is even argued that there are proven links between the use of certain pesticides and the incidence of impotence (Hodson, 1977).[2] The often deleterious effects of drugs generally is now receiving popular coverage, but it could be more sharply focused on this particular problem. It is now estimated that possibly as many as forty-five drugs regularly prescribed by doctors can render men incapable of normal erection. These include antidepressants, tranquillizers, barbiturates, antihistamines and various bromides. Most drugs that are used to control high blood pressure can cause erectile problems; it sounds alarmist, but one report maintains that as many as 41 per cent of those who are so treated are rendered impotent (Hodson, 1977).

Other physical factors, which range from organic disease and the post-operative repercussions of surgery to the more remediable effects of nicotine, obesity and poor diet, can all take their toll. There is a wide variety of possible physical causes (see especially Mudd, 1974), and it is essential that before any treatment is given or recommended as many as possible are eliminated from consideration. This, of course, requires a very thorough examination, which must include some account of the patient's medical history. Sometimes this can be rather difficult: partly because the subject may not be completely forthcoming on some matters; partly because of the sheer diversity of possible causes; and not least of all because any physical factor that is identified may turn out to be only one of many contributory causes.

The problem of just how to distinguish possible physical causes from possible psychological ones is vitiated by certain sets of assumptions. There is a marked tendency 'in the trade' to regard most secondary impotence as psychological in origin. Such assumptions have good clinical support. But indirectly, this gives rise to the complementary tendency to underplay the possibilities of physical disorder and particularly the role of drugs as causal factors in sexual dysfunction. No one is suggesting that this is part of some deeply laid medical conspiracy; but it is difficult to avoid the suspicion that the profession has a well attested investment in the efficacy of drug therapy generally and is consequently reluctant to admit that it can have untoward — and certainly undetected — side-effects. Patients rarely seem to be told about such effects[3] for two main reasons. First, it is rather doubtful in some cases whether the doctors themselves are aware of these specific potentialities of certain drugs; and, second, where they are known, non-communication may be rationalized in terms of clinical expediency. After all, if the patient is informed that the drugs he is prescribed are likely to cause impotence, what is a mere physiological possibility can be transposed into a physical actuality. By a subtle interpretive process, the expected may become the experienced.

The impotence problem has another 'physical' dimension which is certainly given insufficient attention in much of the literature, and which may well be a crucial factor in any dysfunctional syndrome. This concerns the attitudes of the subject to the physical characteristics of both himself and his partner. The liberated literature on positional and orgasm-enhancing techniques has to assume the presence of unalloyed physical attraction, even for ageing couples. The male, regardless of his own physical deficiencies, may require something more appealing in his partner. Of course, his own sense of deficiency may be a prime source of inhibition with a younger woman, and this will only serve to increase his sexual anxieties. There is evidence of considerable sexual difficulties among older men engaged in group sex where both younger men and younger women are able to make the obvious physical comparisons (Bartell, 1971). On the other hand, men not infrequently expect something more of their partners than they do of themselves. Inconsistent as it may seem, they do not find it easy to overlook the wrinkled bellies and the sagging breasts. Even genuine affection cannot always bridge the gulf between what was once desirable and what is now desired. It is hardly a consolation to be told by the therapists to 'fantasize and imagine model girls'.[4] Admittedly, the models have nothing the partner has not, but usually the distribution is a little different.

A more specific variant of the partner problem concerns the possible transmission of real or imagined infections. Again, this is a matter that tends to be minimized in the literature. The manuals, not unusually, concentrate on extremes. There is often some information about specific venereal diseases together with general advice about personal hygiene, but little about the more common sexually transmitted diseases such as thrush and *trichamonis vaginalis*. These fungoidal and parasitic infections are not particularly harmful, but they can be decidedly unpleasant and very persistent. They are usually accompanied by itching, perhaps a localized rash, and offensive genital discharges and odours, especially in the female. There is a tendency to dismiss these as minor irritations which can easily be treated by modern preparations. But this is not always the case. Some drugs and broad-spectrum anti-fungoidal creams work with some people but they are not *permanently* effective with all. It is now fairly widely accepted that such infections are on the increase (see for example Rorvik and Devlin, 1975, p. 196). This has been variously attributed to a number of possible causes ranging from the widespread use of the contraceptive pill to the near-universal adoption of tight nylon underwear.[5] Whatever the causes, such factors do not exactly inspire sexual confidence. The male may find the prospects rather disheartening; intercourse becomes an anxiety, and the exotica of oral-genital contact even more daunting. It does seem at least possible that a combination of apprehension and repugnance may induce sexual problems. Of course, one may well ask if this sort of bacterial inconvenience should really deter the full-blooded male? Whatever became of the daredevil 'Don't-care-if-I-do-go-blind' spirit of the intrepid brothel-goer?[6] Yet it may be precisely this fear of *direct* contact that is just one factor in the recent overshadowing of conventional prostitution by the rising personal massage trade.

From this discussion, we can see how very easy it is to move from the purely physical — which in this context has a very limited meaning — to the psychological. It is extremely difficult to divorce physical factors, attributes or whatever from the attitudes that they generate. And, as we shall see, it is equally difficult to determine priority sequences; does the factor generate the attitude, or does the attitude affect the factor? And if, in fact, the interaction is reciprocal, in what ways and in what situations does it operate?

SENSUALITY-DEPRIVATION THEORIES

Here again we have to consider what are basically physical factors which are said to impinge upon and shape our attitudes, but in this case they are very specifically focused.

It has been seriously argued that the absence of bodily contact, particularly in the formative years, affects the nature of our interactive capacities in later life. In other words, if our mothers had fondled us longer, we would be nicer people. By what is largely a 'read-back' method, it is contended that those who are withdrawn or who tend to exhibit anti-social behaviour are likely to be those who have been deprived of this tactility-enhancing contact in infancy. Complementarily, it is maintained that all is never lost; even in later life, our tactile sensitivities can be restored and used to our advantage. 'Touch' as a form of alleviative treatment can still be effective for would-be delinquents and tired businessmen alike (see for example Leidloff, 1977).

There is nothing really new in this approach; it has long been part of the theoretical apparatus of the social anthropologists (for instance Mead, 1954), who have naively entertained the a-functionalist notion that what appears to work for primitives can be successfully adopted by advanced societies.[7] A social practice is effective because it is a part of a viable complex of practices. But what 'works' in one context does not necessarily work in another. More 'intimate' and permissive modes of child-rearing are a characteristic of some primitive societies where public order is a function of social rather than legal sanctions. But it cannot be simplistically assumed that they can be directly adapted to the needs of advanced systems, where the problems of control are infinitely more complex and the traditional prerequisites just do not exist. In cases where 'progressive' methods have been tried by educationists for social reasons they have rarely met with academic success. The exception has been in situations where there were small classes, caring parents and exceptional teachers (see Tribe, 1975, p. 143). Innovation of any kind, whether in general or in specifically sexual education, must take account of prevailing norms and values.

The development of tactile sensitivity either as an institutionalized pastime or as an informal activity, is held to be both psychologically and socially therapeutic. Proximity sessions, of a formal or informal nature, in which bodily contact is either stipulated or encouraged is seen as an aid to social harmony and understanding. To explore the body is to explore the interstices of the human condition. It is all a very serious business, especially in its carefully commercialized Esalen forms, where it is pursued as a highly lucrative — and, of course, socially responsible — enterprise. The most famous of their self-improvement centres at Big Sur in California caters for some 1,500 people each summer. When not massaging one another's bodies and psyches, they participate in a wider variety of outdoor activities on a relentlessly healthy diet (Leo, 1977). Esalen has spawned a number of imitations all concerned with physical and psychic health. Their evangel is reasonably clear: if we all huddled a little closer together, the world would be a much better place.

A similar message is implied in recent trends towards social osculation (Morrow, 1977). Public kissing is variously regarded in different cultures as a sign of friendship, as among Arabs; as offensive and unsanitary, in Japan; or even as an intimation of impending death, as in the Mafia. Evidence suggests that kissing as a social gesture is now on the increase. Perhaps the inspiration for the current outbreak comes largely from show business via the media. 'Increased kissing is part of the general inflation of intimate signals. We kiss people we used to hug, and hug people we used to shake hands with, and shake hands with people we used to nod to' (Murray Davis, sociologist, quoted in Morrow, 1977). Etiquette and good neighbourliness demand it. The community spirit is in and social isolationism is out. Not to kiss or hug is not to relate, and not to relate is tantamount to enjoying personal privacy.

Touch therapy is hardly a threat to civilization, and is probably not without some value. The thing that detracts from taking its advocates too seriously must be its underlying assumption that fundamental relationships can be changed by expressive tactility. It may well be that one can get to know others more quickly this way, but to know is not necessarily to like, and to touch is not necessarily to caress — a fact well known even to the most unenterprising sadist. Touch therapy is not going to change society, even if it does affect the attitudes of some individuals. It follows, therefore, that the deprivation of tactile awareness, as the devotees understand it, is not exactly fatal. It may just be that some people are sexually inadequate because they lack tactile sensitivity, but it is highly debatable whether this can be regarded as any kind of general explanation, or whether touch therapy can be considered a sexual panacea.

Psychological Theories

The majority of current theorists adopt what is essentially a psychological approach to sexual problems, and increasing numbers of general practitioners and psychiatrists are now operating in the sex therapy field. It is now commonly accepted in medical practice that, where possible, the 'whole' person should be treated, and this is particularly true in the case of sexual dysfunction. In diagnosis, it is possible only rarely to distinguish the obvious physical manifestations from probable psychological influences. Even where there is known organic disease or physical deficiency, these will almost invariably have psychological repercussions. The interaction between the mind and the body is one of inextricable complexity. Indeed, purists might argue that 'mind' and 'body' are only artificially separable. In themselves, they are merely convenience terms, and perhaps the term 'mind-body' might be preferable.

Broadly speaking, psychological theories of impotence are related to general personality defects, or to specific or conjectural factors in the subject's personal biography. Both approaches tend to assume that, where the subject is educable, the hypothesized causes of dysfunction can be effectively neutralized if not eradicated altogether.

Recourse to personality factors as an explanation of dysfunction has to be frustratingly vague, yet the texts are replete with allusions of this kind. 'It is probable, though not certain, that impotence is more frequent in men of neurotic personality (anxious, tense, insecure; liable to phobias, insomnia and mild depression; lacking in confidence, obsessional, hypochondriacal and so on). This type of personality is partly inherited' (Gillan and Gillan, 1976, p. 116). The terms that are being used here — neurotic, phobic, obsessional, etc. — are scientifically meaningless. They are simply inferential categories based on specific experiences. They *describe* certain features of some men's behaviour, but they *explain* nothing. A man may be phobic or obsessional or whatever about a very narrow range of conditions, his appearance, his work or his health, or even about singular things such as his car, his hair or his fingernails. We must be careful not to confuse individualism with idiosyncracy. But if we are going to insist on regarding him as neurotic about any one of these, we must beware of extrapolating from the particular to the general and labelling him a 'neurotic personality'. And all this tells us nothing about *why* this person has developed these traits in the first place. To argue that sexual dysfunction or anything else derives from personality factors is simply to push the problem a little further away. It is a non-answer at one remove.

Purported explanations in terms of personality are usually related to learning processes. It is assumed that most sexual problems do not derive from some kind of physiological deficiency but are psychogenic, that is to say, psychological in origin. Although no adequate statistics are available, it is believed that the majority of those who experience sexual difficulties are biologically normal (Gillan and Gillan, 1976, p. 73) and therefore have the capacity for sexual re-education. The psychological barriers to satisfactory sexual activity are then often traced to what are regarded as faulty learning processes. Sexual ignorance is seen as the key problem: ignorance, first of all, of our basic physiology and its functions. How many girls, we are asked,[8] have viewed their labia in a mirror, that is from the male perspective? How many men have explored the sensitivity of the frenum? Second, ignorance of sexual techniques is cited, and — especially if we are unemancipated women — ignorance of our sexual potential. Almost invariably, these problems are seen as the inevitable result of undersirable restraints in our childhood. Prejudiced parents told us sex was evil, and refused open discussion of the subject. Sexual curiosity was regarded as unbecoming in healthy citizens, and genital investigation was positively discouraged. Our tumescent urges went unheeded, and their suppression, we are told, has given rise to the inhibited and guilt-ridden individuals we are today. And to complicate matters even further, this approach to the elucidation of sexually related problems is often aided by the doubtful specificities of psychoanalysis.

Just how do psychoanalytic theories (and the plurality of such theories should be stressed) see the sexual development of the individual? First, they are not too sure about the earliest formative influences. *Pre*-natal factors are by no means discounted. The comforting sense of uterine snugness and security and the great primary trauma of birth when the experience is shattered are all part of the theoretical stock-in-trade of psychoanalysis. Indeed, the *avant-garde* have gone even further. The psyche is now being probed by therapists who see the real answer to our problems in terms of some previous life-experience. Reincarnation therapy, which hypothesizes that the root of our problems, sexual and otherwise, lies in one of our earlier incarnations, pushes the unknown to the ultimately unknowable. Reincarnation-oriented therapy is undoubtedly on the increase in the United States, where more and more practitioners are using standard techniques, including meditation and hypnosis, to re-acquaint patients with their previous lives. It is even suspected that the past life movement is actually cashing in on the current disillusionment with conventional therapies (see *Time*, 3 October 1977). However bizarre and attractive as such ideas may be, they are not endorsed by the majority of practitioners.[9]

In general, psychoanalytic theory divides the early years of an individual into four main stages of development. Each stage overlaps and carries its own powerful forms of sexual experience, and helps to shape the subsequent psycho-sexual 'character' of the person concerned.[10] The first stage is marked by oral gratification, and the oral 'type' — who never quite outgrows this stage — may well develop into an amiable, sensually indulgent individual who is probably prone to obesity and coronory thrombosis.

If, on the other hand, the infant has been deprived, it is hypothesized that he may develop into a querulous and resentful person who is permanently at odds with the world. The dawning awareness of his mother is regarded as crucial at this stage, but the secret apparently is in the correct use of her natural resources. 'There is no experience quite as stabilising as *good* breast-feeding' (Coltart and Williams, 1975, p. 34).

The second, or anal, stage involves the imposition of discipline and control. We are told that one possible legacy of this stage is that some people may be left with a strange residue of conflicts:[11] perhaps they will be strongly opinionated, hating to be in the wrong; alternatively, they may be miserly with an inordinate desire to dominate others. This is said to derive from an infant's reluctance to part with his faeces, to the despair of its mother. We are even assured that this 'miserliness' may have certain positive aspects and find vocational expression in later years in the managing of banks or the inspecting of taxes (Coltart and Williams, 1975, p. 39). Again, it hardly needs to be stressed that this kind of assertion has the same unassailable unprovability that is a characteristic of so much psychoanalytical writing. Children pass through this stage when they are about two or three years of age. If they then have to recourse to therapists as adults, possibly in connection with some sexual problem, they usually find it quite impossible to recall anything about this period beyond the vaguest impressions. But if they are sufficiently susceptible, and their need for an explanation is powerful enough, they can often be influenced by high-sounding 'interpretations' of their unremembered experiences.

At about four or five years of age children are said to enter the third stage of their development, the phallic or genital stage. Boys are preoccupied with the task of maintaining the 'safety' of their penises, while little girls are concerned with the fact that they do not appear to have them. It is assumed by some psychotherapists that 'in their secret sex lives [they have been] masturbating for years already' (Coltart and Williams, 1975, p. 41). It is in this stage, we are told, that children assume their ultimate sexual orientations; unconscious choices are made as to whether the individuals concerned will gravitate towards heterosexuality or homosexuality. Even the tendencies towards various kinds of sexual perversions may also be generated at this time (Freud, 1923). In short, it is hypothesized that in these very early formative years children will 'fix' their true sexual identities. It is also during this period that children are said to develop heterosexual desires for the relevant parent, and would actually like to rid themselves of their 'rivals', the opposite parent. Indeed, they find it increasingly frustrating that this wish cannot be realized, and that the whole traumatic process tends to go unrecognized by either parent.

Subsequently, in the latency period that follows before the onset of puberty, the seeming indifference of most children to the implications and attractions of sexuality, and their uniform preoccupation with such harmless pursuits as reading and games, are attributed to the massive repression that has taken place following the inner conflicts of the genital stage. Learning and sport, indeed 'innocence' itself, are seen as forms of sublimation. By this time children's incestuous longings and their patricidal-matricidal fervour have become lost to memory, except of course for those unmentionable urges that later, in their pre-waking moments, catch them unawares. Hence a veritable theology has arisen on the interpretation of dreams for Freudian devotees (cf. Freud, 1900, and Hadfield, 1954). The adult with the presenting symptoms is usually blissfully ignorant of these critical childhood experiences, but — according to psychoanalytical lore — they can often be dredged up from a reluctant unconscious by means of the appropriate techniques. This is all part of the discipline's mystique.

An early discussion of Freud's shows how he attempted to apply these general theoretical ideas to the specific problem of male impotence (see Freud, 1912 and 1930). In doing so, we find that his customary psychoanalytical interpretation includes some quite explicit sociological implications. He maintained that his clinical cases exemplified the difficulties that some men have in reconciling their feelings of tenderness towards their mothers with their recurrent sexual urges. He regarded this continuing incompatibility of the sentimental and the sensuous as a characteristic of civilization. It derived from infantile fixations and inhibited adolescent drives. Civilized society imposed moral constraints. It tried to regulate sexual activity and ensure behavioural conformity by conventional codes of conduct. This might be necessary for the well ordered society, but it was a denial of man's natural inclinations. And the suppression of these normal physical urges brought inevitable operational problems. By implication, uncivilized man was sexually liberated, but civilized man was psychologically emasculated. He lived his life in bio-social confusion. In fact, Freud found that many of his patients could realize their sexuality only with women whom they considered morally or intellectually inferior, i.e. less 'civilized' than themselves. He concluded that potency problems are therefore endemic to civilized society, which inculcates contradictory norms.

This general Freudian model, however, is not without its critics. The transition from stage to stage, during which any individual may become fixated and suffer distortions in their psycho-sexual development, has not always stood up well to experimental validation (note the critical article by Gwynne-Jones, 1976). Freud clung to some views with stubborn tenacity. For example, he held that most, if not all, his female patients had been seduced in childhood by their fathers, though later he recognized that this was probably a fantasy which, nevertheless, had a 'reality' for the patient concerned. It is often supposed that these views may have reflected his clinical preoccupation with middle-class Austrians who had been reared in the sexually repressive atmosphere of the late nineteenth century.

Useful, therefore, as some of his general observations were, especially concerning early sexual exploration and latent infantile responses, their clinical applications have been limited. There appears to be little evidence that psychoanalysis is an adequate technique for the treatment of neurotic conditions, and even less evidence that it is adequate for the modifications of aberrations in sexual behaviour. In fact, some authorities argue that the opposite is the case (see Eysenck and Wilson, 1973).

It is all too easy to find reasons for unusual or eccentric behaviour. In every person's biography there will be a number of experiences that can be 'identified' as the source of the problem. The theoretical favourites tend to be associated with culture in general or with faulty learning processes in particular.

Culture, especially Western culture, is said to impose norms of sexual restraint and reticence with which it is impossible to conform. It may even inculcate negative attitudes towards sex which generate unnecessary feelings of guilt about innocent sexual pursuits. The 'trade' never seem to tire of citing the outmoded strictures of religion in this respect, especially what it regards as the more repressive forms of traditional Christianity (for a typical example of anti-repressive religion literature see Simmons, 1970, chapter 4). Male sexual difficulties are not infrequently related to the ascendancy of the aesthetic Christian ideal, which traditionally elevated celibacy and chastity in its hierarchy of values. More specifically, society may be held responsible for the lack of more innovative measures in sex education. It may have dated policies on such issues as mass contraception and abortion, all of which can influence individual sexual orientations.

Alternatively, the blame may be laid at the door of the transmission agencies themselves, most specifically upon those luckless parents who were unenlightened enough to smack a son's hand which had strayed too near his genitals, or who had remonstrated with a fourteen-year old daughter who argued that 'if you're not on the pill, you can't get a boyfriend' (quoted by Yule, 1978). Progress-defying acts of this kind are often regarded as either ignorant or stupid, and definitely calculated to breed the worst kind of inhibitions in the child. Yet, plausible as it may seem, it is extremely difficult to establish an incontravertible causal connection between disciplinary restrictions and later manifestations of sexual dysfunction. And this is pre-eminently so in the case of impotence.

It is all too easy to attribute male sexual anxieties to the secret struggles of childhood and adolescence. Acts of 'transference' are said to take place, and individuals regress to infantile attitudes that negate or neutralize their current sexual activities, giving rise to an assortment of complexes and neuroses. These may include furtive masturbation, a dread of domineering fathers, castration fears and a sense of guilt when sexual partners are identified with mothers or sisters. Indeed, we are informed that Freud personally cured the composer Gustav Mahler of impotence in *one* therapeutic session by pointing out Mahler's unconscious confusion of his wife with his mother who were both named Marie (Abse, 1974).

This is typically to confuse explanation with cause. It may well be that certain explanations that derive from given psychoanalytical models can be useful in certain cases. This does not demonstrate the validity of the models in general or the specific applications in particular; it merely shows that an explanation that is accepted by a patient — usually when nothing better is forthcoming — can prove to be therapeutically beneficial. But this tells us nothing whatsoever about the *actual* cause of the problem, merely something about the suggestibility of the subject. It is not easy to account for this phenomenon, but it is well attested pragmatically. We are not even sure just why the implantation of certain ideas 'works' in certain circumstances with certain patients; it seems simply adventitious that they do so. Certain childhood experiences are insufficient to explain current sexual difficulties (Kaplan, 1974, pp. 143-5), and, persuasive as such modes of explanation can be, no connections can actually be demonstrated between those early experiences and the dysfunctions they are supposed to have caused.

Psychoanalysis can be a useful adjunct of psychology. But, as some analysts themselves have asserted (see Ryecroft, 1966), it should renounce its theoretical pretensions and confine its attention to the consulting room.

SOCIOLOGICAL THEORIES

Hypothesizing about a given clinical condition, in this case male sexual impotence, usually begins with some implicit notion of abnormality. For simplicity, the issue of abnormality may be seen in three different ways:

(1) as an underlying pathological condition;
(2) as a deviation from a statistical norm;
(3) as a deviation from a culturally desirable ideal.

In practice these criteria may — and often do — overlap, but any sociological theory of impotence tends to put emphasis squarely on the cultural factor. It questions the bases of given cultural norms, and examines the ways in which these are internalized by the individual who then expresses them in subsequent patterns of behaviour.

At the most general level, sexual dysfunction can be

related to circumstantial factors, which tend to generate personal anxieties. In modern society, for example, this can be seen as a function of the industrial process. The tedium of routinized tasks and the repetitive nature of work may bring a depressing sense of alienation. Possibly boredom and disinterestedness are carried over into the personal sphere. Alternatively, perhaps disenchantment with the work situation itself breeds a need for compensatory leisure experience. Sexual problems can certainly arise where there is an obsessive desire to have a good time 'while its still possible'. People try too hard, and over-anxious attempts to maximize sexual experience may ultimately prove to be counter-productive.

In quite different circumstances, i.e. in the complementary world of white-collar responsibilities, the result may be much the same. The unending pressure of work, the lack of time and the preoccupation of unfulfilled office tasks can bring similar problems. Theoretically, this can all be rather loosely related to class factors and the unremitting competitiveness that characterizes capitalistic societies. But perhaps this is too simplistic. These difficulties are not peculiar to the West. Alienation and its attendant problems are probably more a function of industrialization generally than of capitalism in particular.[12] There is no concrete evidence to suggest that the West enjoys a monopoly of sexual dysfunction; and impotence is certainly not a bourgeois conspiracy.

Sociologists, too, are interested in anomic factors. What happens when people lack any sense of meaningful order in society? For a long time, theorists have recognized a breakdown in the old normative structures which do not seem to have been supplanted by anything more certain than a vague ethical neutrality. Nothing is sure any more. To advocate standards, even to hint at the possibility of moral objectivity or self-evident obligations, is to invite scepticism, if not ridicule. Rules of behaviour are intellectually indefensible; discipline is socially *démodé*, if not actually a dirty word.

Not everyone agrees that what has ensued is altogether a bad thing. The codes may have gone, but these have been replaced by the increasing moralization of the individual will. People are said to lead their own lives as long as it 'does not hurt others'. This is arguably the age of increasing political consciousness and social responsibility, but these laudable concerns seem only to be encapsulated in constitutional codes designed to preserve legal order and ensure civic rights. The traditional — often religious — precepts that once informed large areas of personal and even communal practice tend now to be regarded as either undesirable or unattainable ideals. But has this stress on individual interpretation got its weaknesses? Can there be no guideline other than an amorphous and ill-defined social concern?

The uncertainties about social morality can be extended to the question of values associated with social differentiation. It is contended that there was a time when people knew their place, and recognized the values appropriate to their particular situation. This is now regarded as a thing of the past. The old distinctions no longer obtain, and this is especially so in relation to the place of women.

In modern society, there has now been something of a reversal of roles. The patterns of sexual expectation are changing, and we are told that women are assuming a more aggressive stance. This is largely a function of general socio-economic factors, particularly the extension of educational opportunity and the less discriminatory employment practices, which were brought about less by the agitations of the early suffragette movements than by the manpower exigencies of the First World War. The insistent industrial machine requires operators. Women have found a measure of self-expression in comparable work with comparable pay. Complementarily, technology has also come to the aid of women as housewives. Obviously, where women are no longer burdened by large families and have a surfeit of labour-saving gadgetry, domesticity gives way to career aspirations.

Perhaps even more determinate in the case of women are the biological factors: the near-perfection and popularity of conception control techniques, and the easy availability of abortion and sterilization. These are obviously important at several levels, and perhaps, in some ways, their essentiality has been rather generously interpreted. They are necessary aids in the growing world population problem. Equivalently, it can be argued that they are crucial ingredients of the truly free society where both men and women have the right to control their own fertility.

In the sexual stakes, the trump card appears to have been played by Masters and Johnson with their 'discovery' that women have greater orgasmic capacities than men. It is claimed that sexual ascendancy has passed to the female. Men, it is argued, are in retreat. They have been socialized in terms of a sexual dominance which their biology is unable to support (Bowskill and Linacre, 1977A). Their sexual potential is refractorily limited. So the initiative is said to have transferred to the traditionally 'weaker sex', who are now able to exploit it to the disadvantage of resentful males. Men now find themselves unable to meet the rising expectations of female sexual demand. The old stigma of female frigidity is being overshadowed by the emergent phenomenon of male impotence.

This interpretation of apparent trends seems to be held by a number of authorities in the field. Robert Murphy, for example, argues that *mutual* sexual gratification has set up anxieties in men that inhibit their performance as lovers: 'every revolution has its casualties. Impotent men are the major casualties of the sexual revolution' (reported by Silverberg, 1978).

The validity of this thesis is still an open question. We have already examined some of the orgasmic implications (chapter 1), which seriously qualify some of its main contentions. And we have also shown (chapter 2) that, given the female capacity for repeated intercourse, there is no firm evidence that this is being aggressively exploited to the embarrassment of the male. Capacity does not equal libido. We have yet to ascertain whether this new-found clitoral potential has actually altered the balance of their respective sexual drives.

Sociological perspectives, in most cases, complement rather than contradict psychological interpretations. Freud inclined to the view that successful sexuality depended upon a return to 'nature', or at least to a discovery of one's 'true', unsocialized nature. Sociologists tend to desert Freud at this point. Instead, they emphasize not the recovery of one's essential nature, but the making of one's *own* nature. On this interpretation, nature is relative; it is largely a cultural product. The raw materials are given in our physical makeup, but they are developed and shaped by social interaction. This orientation is essentially existential. In a sense, we are all 'becoming', and we cannot, therefore, discover or recover our true selves because self-hood is fluid and ever-changing. We are not what we were yesterday, and will be different again tomorrow. Action and interaction alter the 'we' that we are. It follows, on this view, that there is no 'set' sexuality, no pre-ordained sexual roles.[13] There is neither homosexuality nor heterosexuality, nor in one sense is there male or female. All sexual meanings become negotiable. For sexual purposes, we can choose our own sex, determine our own sexuality, be what we want to be. This may all make a kind of biological nonsense, but — with serious reservations — it has some interesting cultural implications. It can be fairly assumed that it has ideological undertones, and that it stems from the current egalitarian obsession with innate human capacities which can be realized only in the rightly ordered society.

The sociological approach to sexual dysfunction focuses attention on received social values and consequently on the actors rather than the act, and the situations in which they operate. To its detriment, sociology tends to minimize biological factors, but it is surely correct to argue that man's biology is insufficient to equip him for social life, and that a socialization process of considerable complexity is required if social adaptation and integration are to take place with any reasonable degree of success. The process is, of course, unavoidable. There is a modern tendency to see it as restrictive and inhibiting. The family and the educational institutions are sometimes regarded as oppressive agents of control which force the young into predetermined moulds, the implication being that, if only people were allowed to find their own way, unfettered by conditioning mechanisms, they would somehow develop richer personalities and, arguably, healthier sex lives. This assumes that there is an inner, inviolable 'self' to be discovered, a 'nature' as yet unrealized. Sociologists, on the other hand, would tend to emphasize the existential realities. The essential self is something of an unknown quantity. But what can be asserted with some confidence is that we are all capable of some change and adaptation through the everyday process of social interaction.

'Correct' socialization, then, is seen as a means towards social maturity, an extension of a person's social roles and an expansion of his ability to appreciate the role definitions of other people. In this way he is initiated into the evaluations of the particular culture of which he is a part. This involves a dialectic between the individual and society. He actively participates in a process of adjustment in which — in the situation under discussion — he gradually acquires patterns of sexual behaviur of which society approves. In a sense, by his very presence he helps to 'make' society, but society and its values also make him. It was here before he arrived, and it will presumably still be here when he leaves. The impression he makes during his relatively short stay will probably be minimal, and even this will be a reflection of the cultural system that he has inherited.

A person's early, or primary, socialization is important — as the psychologists rightly point out — but his secondary socialization into the meanings of what it is to be 'manly' or 'virile' may well be crucial to his subsequent sexual behaviour. These are inculcated not only through the screening activities of the family and the initial educational process, but also through the influences of the peer group value system. These are crucial ingredients in a culture that 'constructs' a given sexual ideology. Cultures perpetuate the prevailing sexual images and decide standards of beauty, modes of attraction, and what are and what are not acceptable levels of performance.

It is at this point that biology and sociology tend to part company when they should be realizing their complementarity. Sociology recognizes that we are all subject to given physiological mechanisms, but it insists that sexuality — and, more importantly, the *expression* of that sexuality — are conditioned not simply by biological imperatives, but also by the social meanings with which they are endowed. This necessarily involves a change in perspective. The emphasis shifts from the act itself to the *total context* in which the act is expressed. For many, this can make all the difference to the question of sexual functionality and dysfunctionality.

7. Sex Therapies

Some of the most extensive research findings in the area of sexual dysfunction are those of Masters and Johnson.[1] As we have already seen, they distinguish between *primary* impotence, where the male has apparently never been able to have intercourse, and *secondary* impotence, where there is a history of at least one successful act of intercourse but where the subject is now no longer able either to obtain or to maintain an erection. The occasional failure that some men have owing to tiredness or alcoholic indulgence or whatever is not classified as secondary impotence unless it leads to a persistent failure syndrome. It might, therefore, be useful at this stage of the discussion to summarize briefly these findings, and the causal explanations that derive from them.

Taking primary impotence first: in the eleven years prior to the publication of their book Masters and Johnson (1970) had treated 32 males in this category. Of these, 22 were not married while undergoing therapy, but many of them had a record of unsuccessful marriage owing to their sexual inadequacy. Masters and Johnson maintain that there was usually no clear single reason for the condition; in any one case, there was a complex of causes, both social and psychological. However, they did identify a number of factors:

(1) In 3 cases, there was evidence of incestuous overtures by their mothers during the patients' early years.

(2) In 6 cases, there had been youthful homosexual attachments, and with some men there was still some uncertainty about their 'true' sexual natures. Presumably, this ambiguity of orientation affected their sexual performance.

(3) In 4 cases, the men had had disastrous initial experiences with prostitutes, and their humiliation had been so traumatic that sex had become something to be both feared and avoided.

It was recognized by Masters and Johnson that this did not constitute an inviolable rule; some men who had experienced very severe sexual traumas did not become impotent, and there was no simple explanation for this.

(4) The researchers insisted that the single most common factor was strict adherence to certain forms of religious training. It was hypothesized that observation of taboos combined with considerable misinformation really lay behind their condition. What cannot be easily explained is why untold numbers of other men subjected to the same or similar modes of religious instruction respond quite normally. It would seem that the 'fault' does not necessarily lie with the religious teaching as such, but either with its inculcation by particular parents/teachers, or with its idiosyncratic interpretation by the subjects themselves.

Next, there is the more common problem of secondary impotence. In this area, similar factors were identified by Masters and Johnson.

(1) There was some relationship between impotence and premature ejaculation; this showed in 63 of the 213 cases that were treated. In most instances, the patients had a history of ejaculatory difficulties before the onset of secondary impotence.

(2) Drinking was also a very common factor. Some 35 patients — mostly businessmen — were treated whose initial failures had almost certainly been precipitated by over-indulgence of alcohol.

(3) More amorphously, Masters and Johnson associated impotence and sexual insecurity with dominance of the family by either the father or mother. They obviously regarded this as an incorrect form of socialization. In 23 of their patients, they saw examples of where they felt demanding and disapproving parents had undermined the sexual confidence of their children. They also detected a tendency for mother-dominated boys to become wife-dominated men, thus perpetuating the pattern, and detracting even further from their sense of masculinity.

This has to be an extremely tenuous hypothesis. There are no adequate measures of what it means to be 'demanding' and 'disapproving'. We cannot assess the influence of 'dominance' with any certainty. It could equally well be argued that mother-dominated men tend to rebel against their childhood experience, or even — on another analysis — become homosexuals. Without more intensive investigation, this line of Masters and Johnson must be regarded as cognitively unsatisfactory.

(4) Again, homosexuality in the formative years is regarded as important. This applied to 21 patients, and what is regarded as particularly interesting is that in each case their first sexual activities had been of a homosexual kind. Some commentators have remarked that 'the man whose first mature sexual experience is homosexual appears to be marked by it, even though he switches to heterosexual lovemaking' (Belliveau and Richter, 1971, p. 139).

Yet again, this is an unverifiable hypothesis, and at best is simply impressionistic. What Freud would have made of this is hardly a matter of surmise; he argued that early male sexual experiences were often homosexual. Certainly some societies, notably ancient Thebes and Sparta, recognized it as part of the young male's sexual development, prior to compulsory heterosexual marriage (see Flaceliere, 1973).

(5) The religious factor is cited in 26 of the 213 cases. Their distribution in terms of the type of religious organization concerned immediately suggests that this hypothesis should be treated with some reserve, 6 were Jewish, 11 were Catholic, 4 fundamentalist Protestant and 5 were from mixed marriages. The distribution is therefore quite wide, and does not point incontravertibly to any one particular religious persuasion. It also means that some 187 of the patients with presumably non-inhibiting religious upbringings were nevertheless having marked erectile problems.

The points made in relation to those suffering from primary impotence apply equally well here. It makes reductionist nonsense to try to relate the incidence of a problematical phenomenon such as impotence to any one variable, particularly when that variable — in this case, religion — is a ubiquitous fact of human society.

Rightly or wrongly, religion is often regarded as a principal factor in faulty socialization. The aim of some sexual re-education is to convince the patient of the invalidity of the religious prohibitions that circumscribe sexual behaviour. Once the myths and misconceptions have been dealt with, it is assumed that he will soon be on the road to recovery. But we can see from the actual results that the therapies are rather less suspect than the analysis.

Useful as the work of Masters and Johnson has been at

the investigatory and therapeutic levels, its theoretical and interpretive suggestions are far from satisfactory. They maintained that only seven of their patients had physical problems, and insisted that the real explanation had to be sought — perhaps rightly — in psycho-social factors. But here there are frustrating uncertainties. What one does for a latent homosexual businessman from a demanding religious home is anybody's guess. It remains for us to see how well the therapies actually work.

There is no one kind of sex therapy. They come in various guises, and emanate from schools that represent different theoretical positions. These are usually reflected in the kinds of treatment that are given. Therapists are generally agreed on what therapy *is*, but there are often conflicting opinions as to how it should be practised. The aims of sex therapy are reasonably clear, but what is in dispute is just how these aims should be operationalized. At the most general level, we can see that, by the use of a number of reasonably well established techniques, therapists hope to modify or 'correct' certain kinds of detrimental sexual behaviour in their patients. The techniques themselves, and sometimes their respective rationales, however, are still the sources of some debate. Basically, sex therapies are directed towards the resolution of sexual difficulties. But whether the primary objective is the establishment of good sexual relations or the facilitation of good sexual performance — which has narrower connotations — is still uncertain. The two clearly go together, but they are not inseparable.

At a more particular level, the aim of some sex therapy is concerned not so much with *what* is being done but *to whom* it is being done. The intention may be to alter the focus of sexual attention rather than the performance itself. For instance, the paedophiliac may operate very efficiently with young children and experience neither erectile difficulties nor residues of remorse, but cultural norms demand the realignment of his sexual concern (see Gagnon, 1977, p. 365). Therapy therefore will be required not to cure sexual inadequacy, but to effect some kind of redirection of his sexual attentions.

We can see here that society, in general, is pursuing conflicting aims. While certain categories of sexual behaviour are still proscribed as deviant, there is increasing pressure to recognize more sexual minorities. Male and female homosexuals are to be accepted; fetishism and transvestitism together with sado-masochism are to be seen as 'comprehensible' sexual sub-cultures. There are even serious moves to convince society of the desirability — almost the nobility — of paedophilia. What was once objectionable is now being tolerated. Distinctions are becoming blurred. What were deviations are now known euphemistically as variations. In a qualified sense, a 'whatever-turns-you-on' ethos prevails.

It is not surprising that the overriding intention of modern sex therapy is to establish sexual competence. This, in turn, improves sexual performance, which presumably gives greater or renewed satisfactions. This is all consistent with the permissive climate of opinion in society. Attitudes are relaxing, the old inhibitions are going. What matters is *success* — particularly sexual success. Whatever the object of desire happens to be, that desire should be realized without difficulty. And as these difficulties can most probably be induced by the stirrings of guilt, therapy may have to be directed towards the eradication of moral unease. Hang-ups must give way to a cultivated hedonism.

There is yet another sense in which society's aims appear to be inconsistent. While supporting the rights of sexual minorities, it is — simultaneously — moving away from a stress on collective goals to an emphasis on personal standards. Group rights are applauded, but, at the same time, conduct is seen as problematic only when it becomes a problem for *individuals*. The consenting adult conscience is now said to constitute the moral baseline for social behaviour (Gagnon, 1977). In practice, it is difficult to see how these can easily be separated. To some extent, the individual conscience can usually be seen to reflect the norms of some collectivity or other, if not of the consensus itself.

Perhaps one further preliminary point should be made. Sex therapies treat sexual dysfunction, but perceptions of what sexual dysfunction is have changed over time. For example, in the past, for a woman to be inorgasmic was considered to be in no way exceptional. In societies where pregnancy is the primary aim of sexual intercourse, the question of female satisfaction may be largely incidental. It is a bonus that is thought desirable, but not essential.[2] The present emphasis on sex for itself indicates a preoccupation with achieving sexual satisfaction rather than facilitating procreation. With modern contraceptive techniques, society can now write new sexual scripts. In this changing context, early ejaculation becomes redefined as *premature* ejaculation, and the condition of female 'frigidity' becomes implicitly the responsibility of the male who has failed in his task as lover. Complementarily, there may be a de-emphasis on coitus, as such, and a subsequent stress on alternative — especially oral-genital — modes of satisfaction. For some women, for instance, this has been reduced to personal masturbation. They are being urged to discover the potentialities of their own bodies (Hite, 1977). This can even be done on a communal basis if they wish; some therapists are actually providing masturbation classes for the more adventurous. Of course, vibrators are the in-thing. When surrendering to the indescribable ecstacies of the electric toothbrush, who needs men? Sexual monism has become the *reductio ad absurdum* of the erotic *avant-garde*.

Sex therapy is not, strictly, a modern phenomenon. As

we have already seen, many primitive and ancient societies were concerned not only with matters of fertility — always a pre-occupying issue in agrarian systems — but also with the question of potency itself, and devised various rituals and charms to ensure its continuance (see Ryley-Scott, 1970). The beginnings of sex therapy can be traced to the belief in love incantations and hopeful assumptions about the efficacy of love philtres. These practices could sometimes be deadly: Aristotle records how a woman in ancient Greece was brought before the judges accused of killing her lover with a love philtre. When they were not dangerous, they might simply be ridiculous, such as hanging crocodile testicles over the nuptial bed in Java when an elderly man married a young girl (Simons, 1970, p. 61).

But modern sex therapy is of quite a different order. Apart from the dubious theoretical underpinnings of psychoanalysis, it can now be said to have a scientific basis. Cognitive pretensions have given way to empirical validity. Its operations therefore merit closer examination.

According to some of its most redoubtable protagonists, modern sex therapy is 'the treatment of sexual problems, based on scientific foundations [which] takes the form of reassurance, education and carefully designed recommendations' (Gillan and Gillan, 1976, p. 1). What is stressed here is that sexual dysfunction is a *problem,* not an illness. Therefore, the medical model of the passive patient who dutifully accepts the treatment and advice of his doctor is not really applicable to the situation. The medical model assumes the wisdom of the doctor, and the effectiveness of the treatment, regardless of the subjective uncertainties of the patient. The therapeutic model, on the other hand, assumes the positive and intelligent co-operation of the patient in an effort to effect a cure. The therapist, therefore, acts as educator rather than a medical authority. It is, of course, duly recognized that the dysfunction in question may be directly related to organic factors, in which case it will be referred to the appropriate agencies. But the underlying presupposition is that in most instances the causes are likely to be of a psycho-social nature. In short, sex therapy seeks by the use of selected techniques to modify or rectify sexual responses that are characterized as problems. The degree of success, in any particular case, will depend on the correct application of those techniques and the ability to convince the patient of their therapeutic potential.[3]

Modern sex therapy is normally associated with behaviour therapy.[4] The fundamental postulate of this approach is that neurotic disorders are simply faulty behaviour patterns which have been induced by traumatic or inappropriate learning experiences, and are therefore potentially modifiable through retraining (see Mackay, 1976).

Some modern therapists make a fine distinction between behaviour therapy and sex therapy (primarily Kaplan, 1974, pp. 202ff.). Behaviour therapy is regarded as primarily an office-based operation in which patients are treated in rather artificial clinical situations. Sex therapy, on the other hand, aims to make the patients their own therapists. This is achieved by following out specific tasks with the patients in suitable environments. These tasks consist mainly of particular sexual acts which would be difficult and unnatural under clinical conditions. They are carried out as part of a carefully organized programme in conducive surroundings, either in the patients' own homes or, sometimes, in a local hotel.[5] It has been argued that behaviour therapy has not enjoyed a great deal of success in relation to sexual dysfunction, and that its reputation is more impressive in the field of sexual variations. But sex therapy, on the other hand, is said to have been very effective when applied to the area of dysfunction (Kaplan, 1974, p. 209). This kind of argument is valid provided one accepts the somewhat artificial distinctions. Behaviour therapy and sex therapy are both rooted in the same theoretical principles; they can be distinguished by their techniques, but both are concerned with very similar overall strategies. In effect, modern sex therapy should probably be considered a form or extension of behaviour therapy.

The development of the behavioural school is different from — and, in some ways, is a reaction to — the more psychoanalytically oriented who maintain that the problem as presented is really an indication of a more profound personality disturbance. But the difference is not so much at the explanatory level; after all, views about faulty socialization, traumatic experiences and personality disturbances can, with a little theoretical contortionism, be safely reconciled. The difference of approach really lies in the operative assumptions that underly their respective methodologies. Whereas the psychoanalysts seek to remove the patient's defences and facilitate an inner awareness, behaviour therapists attempt to modify observable abnormalities by direct manipulation.

Where sexual problems are thought to be amenable to psychoanalytical techniques, it often involves lengthy and expensive treatment in order to identify the 'true' cause of the problem. In contrast, the behaviour therapists are more direct in their approach. They are primarily concerned not with hypothesized causes, but with the treatment of the immediate symptoms. Causes *are* important, *if* they can be known. Using psychoanalytical methods, the reconnaisance can be long and inconclusive, whereas behavioural methods can often produce quite rapid results for the patient. Underlying these different modes of intervention lies a range of assumptions. For the analyst, the symptoms suggest a problem that is deeply rooted in the patient's unconscious mind. This may stem from some traumatic experience in his unremembered youth which has to be teased out by well tried analytical techniques. For the behaviour therapist, the symptoms often suggest a more immediate problem, such as fear of humiliation, which may admit of simpler and quicker amelioration.[6] Such therapies do not necessarily *solve* problems, but they do often overcome the immediate obstacles to effective sexual behaviour. Indeed, the 'real' problem — whatever that may mean — may never actually be discovered. Why a particular man is afraid of women; why he fears humiliation, especially sexual humiliation, may never be known. But, like the intending parachutist who is really afraid of heights, he can be made to jump. Performance does not have to be destroyed by apprehension.

In practice, the distinction between the two approaches is not always clear (a point well made by Cole, 1975, pp. 103-4). Both seek insights; both want to know what the real problems are; and both tend to assume that they are psychodynamic in origin. It is their methods that really distinguish them, and this can be seen most clearly in the issue of direction and non-direction. It is virtually a rule in psychoanalysis that the therapist does not direct or instruct the patient, and may even hesitate to give advice. Even the idea of giving specific sexual tasks may be regarded by some analysts as a form of manipulation of the patient. Instead, there is the pre-supposition that by cathartic interaction and communication with the analyst, a process of self-discovery will take place which will presumably result in a cure. But the success rate for this kind of treatment is not very high, and it sometimes leaves the patient in a state of emotional dependency on the analyst (see Gagnon, 1977, p. 369). In behaviour therapy, however, direction is an essential part of the treatment. The therapist deliberately instructs patients, and expects them to comply, and this has proved to be one of the most effective features of the new approach.

Modern sex therapy owes a great deal to the researches of Masters and Johnson, and most of the techniques that have now been evolved derive very largely from pioneering work that began in the late fifties. First, they made a break with previous traditions by encouraging in their patients a process of sexual re-identification. Those problems that were said to be diseases or neuroses became simply dysfunctions; this implied both something that was not particularly unusual, and something that was probably amenable to the treatment that they were about to offer. This suggestion to patients that the presenting symptoms were merely temporary limitations of their sexual ability created receptive and optimistic attitudes which facilitated treatment procedures. Second, they set out consciously to modify the patients' sexual behaviour by giving them a specific programme of sexual rehabilitation consisting of graded sexual tasks. As William Masters often remarks, the therapy itself does not cure; nature does all the important work. Therapy merely establishes the psychological attitudes whereby the normal physiological responses will occur (quoted by Brecher, 1972, p. 316).

A further assumption that is made by those of the Masters and Johnson school is that preferably therapy should take place in pairs. They feel that, where a male is sexually dysfunctional, it is not only of concern *to* his partner; it may actually have been consciously — or more likely unconsciously — precipitated *by* the partner. It is vital, therefore, that the partner develops the right attitude towards the male condition and learns how to contribute towards its alleviation. It is because a mate is in a unique position either to enhance or destroy the sexual functioning and pleasure of her or his partner that it has become standard practice for many — perhaps most — therapists to work with couples where possible. If the cause of the problem is assumed to be 'dyadic', it must, therefore, be treated accordingly. Complementarily, it is often thought advisable to use dual-sex teams to treat these couples. This is in the Masters and Johnson tradition, and is believed to result in a more balanced and effective implementation of the programme.[7]

Before looking in broad terms at the therapies themselves, one further issue presents itself. With the increase in sex therapy agencies and sex therapy groups, there has been a related increase in sex therapy texts. In fact, the sexual renaissance has gone even further. This proliferation of therapy-oriented literature has been accompanied by the inevitable meta-phenomenon of literature to appraise the literature. Perhaps a discipline has really come of age when it generates its own intra-subject evaluations. Presumably self-criticism is a sign of healthy growth and substantive respectability.

But this raises a problem for the future of sex therapy itself. Should the therapists encourage the use of self-help routines or insist on professionally guided programmes? There are enough manuals available, so what is to stop people from becoming their own therapists?

The professionals' response to this is both guarded and inconsistent. Their philosophy teaches sexual adequacy for all. They are behavioural pragmatists, so they are wedded to whatever works. But they tend to regard themselves as scientists, and many doubt the competence of the half-trained and the untrained, and may actually disparage the efficacy of alternative programmes.

Alternatively, perhaps the two approaches could be successfully combined? After all, Christians can read the Bible for themselves, but they are still enjoined to go to church. Therapists are the priests of the new secular cult of sexual health and their professional livelihood demands that sexual salvation be found only within the sacred community. Theirs is the purity of the faith; they alone are in the true apostolic succession and the self-appointed guardians of the therapeutic gnosis. But perhaps they have only temporal functions in a spiritual order. Their pragmatic concentration on crisis intervention is really a kind of behavioural activism, necessary at the present time. Their theology is often persistently neo-Freudian, and for explanatory purposes many still recourse to the ineffable mysteries of psychoanalytical lore.[8]

In the approach to therapy certain orientational difficulties can also arise. To what extent should the doctor/therapist allow his own sexual proclivities to intrude? Should he, for instance, take the view that, if the patient is not dissatisfied with his own sex life, there is no need for medical intervention? The patient may be a paraphiliac, a homosexual, a deviant of some kind whose views and practices conflict with those of the therapist, and in these circumstances it may be very easy to alienate his sympathies. Of course, the therapist *qua* therapist tries to remain nautral in these matters, but there is bound to remain some underlying opposition of values. There is also the allied situation in which the patient may be seen as a sexual under-achiever; someone who, in the therapist's view, should be enjoying a far more rewarding sex life than he obviously is. The problem this poses is crucial to the value-free posture of sex therapy. If the subject is obviously content with these minimal satisfactions, should he be encouraged to change? Is it the therapist's task to generate a new awareness, to pose questions that no one is asking and to 'solve' difficulties that the patient does not experience? This situation is probably reasonably rare in a 'direct' form, otherwise it is unlikely that the subject would be in consultation with a therapist in the first place. But in tacit forms the issue is really unavoidable. The modification of behaviour is the therapist's *raison d'être*. He must decide whether it should be done, how it should be done, and to what extent it should be done. It is he, *par excellence,* who has implicit notions of what sexual fulfillment ought to be, and he is bound to see the patient's situation in terms of his own idealized models.

The actual therapy programme for male sexual dysfunction varies from therapist to therapist, although they have many features in common. Normally, it begins with a consultation which may have been arranged through the local Marriage Guidance Council, a Family Planning Clinic or some private source — possibly a personal recommendation. Where a man is referred by his doctor it is not unusual to find that impotence was not the presenting symptom or the ostensible reason for the visit. This may have transpired during the discussion; perhaps 'divulged' with some reluctance, or even as a planned 'afterthought'.

The man is interviewed, where possible with his partner, by the therapist, or therapists if a dual-sex team is being used. A complete medical history of the patient will be required and, if necessary, other medical and psychiatric tests or examinations will be made. In this way the therapist will build up a picture of the patient's sexual biography to discover how and when the symptoms first became evident, and in what ways they have been dealt with to date. This picture will then be complemented and even corrected, where possible, by the impressions of the partner, especially if it is a regular partner. Of course, in a number of cases this cannot be done. Perhaps the partner will refuse to co-operate because it is thought to be unnecessary or simply because it is downright embarrassing; in other cases, there may be either a surplus of possible partners to enlist, or no particular partner at all.

This clinical history-taking will probably follow a set pattern, although many therapists allow for an 'open-ended' approach in order to elicit as much information as possible from the patients (see Appendix). The treatment programme itself may be confined to a brief set period in which the patients are seen daily, or it may be extended over a much longer period. This may be carried out in a neutral environment such as a hotel, which allows patients to get away from business and domestic pressures for a while, or it may be conducted in the home itself. Much depends on where the clinic or consulting rooms are located, and even more on the capacity of the patients to afford travelling and hotel expenses in addition to the fees that may be charged. In the United States this has given rise to the allegation that patients are predominantly middle-class, and that we really know comparatively little about the sexual capacities and incapacities of the mass of the people whose situations are not reflected in clinical records.[9]

Some therapists, especially those of the Masters and Johnson school, have fairly rigidly organized programmes which are applied to a variety of different sexual problems. Others are more eclectic in their approach and utilize a wider range of therapeutic techniques depending on the psychodynamics of the case in question. It should perhaps be reiterated that in all modes of treatment the first essential is symptom relief. If this in turn facilitates any kind of conflict resolution in the individual, or between the patient and his partner, it will be considered a desirable and welcome bonus, but it may not necessarily be a precondition of that relief. Other, perhaps deeper, problems may underlie the sexual dysfunction, but it is a *sine qua non* of modern sex therapy that it is possible to treat the symptom regardless of its ultimate cause or causes. Nevertheless, although the primary concern of the therapist is not marital pathology, in much conjoint therapy it is usual to try to encourage the couple to talk through their sexual problems, and these are often inextricably bound up with related marital-domestic issues. Indeed, their relationship may constitute a potentially destructive system, which must be 'interrupted' if it is to be saved. The presupposition here is that, if it can be modified or corrected at one point — in this case, the sexual dimension — this may have beneficial repercussions throughout the mechanism. The idea that if people are happy in bed they are also happy in the kitchen has some cogency. It is almost certainly the case that where they are *not* happy in bed, other niggling domestic issues may assume greater proportions. Obviously, this is not an inviolable rule, but it does seem to accord with much everyday experience.

As a number of different approaches are used by different therapists, a purely descriptive catalogue of the techniques employed would not be particularly rewarding. It is important, therefore, to spend some time discussing the principles underlying the therapies generally, as well as to depict some of the most common procedures themselves. The primary aim of therapy is the restoration of sexual confidence in the patient. This is done by creating what in technical terms is called a non-demanding ambience, that is to say, conditions in which the patient is not required to produce physical responses that are beyond his control. It is vital in these initial stages to minimize his sense of failure, and an intensive programme of sexual re-education is begun with the intention of reducing his *immediate* need to achieve. There is a de-emphasis on performance, especially on performance as measured by orgasm. In removing the psychological pressure to succeed, the therapist hopes that nature will eventually take its course, and normal sexual relations will be resumed.

How is this done? What techniques are employed? Initially, in most treatment programmes a period of sexual abstinence is enjoined. Couples are directed to refrain from sexual contacts until they are told they can do so, and then — as we shall see — these are only permitted on a carefully graded scale.

For general purposes, the Masters and Johnson approach can be regarded as generic, and it would be instructive to follow its general course. Therapists first of all try to ensure that there is no essential conflict of interests in the partners concerned. This necessitates a free exchange of views and opinions, and may involve a 'working-through' of domestic grievances and other parasexual sources of discontent. The airing of these anxieties and disappointments can act as kind of catharsis, and may eventually lead to the partial resolution of certain misconceptions that they have had of their own situations. This kind of exercise seems obvious and even simple in the extreme, but it is not always easy to accomplish. In some circumstances the patient may have only just managed to persuade his or her partner to co-operate, in which case communication may be somewhat circumscribed. In other instances there may appear to be an easy atmosphere, but it becomes obvious to the therapist from the nuances of the conversation that there are certain resentments that are not being voiced. Naturally, this can prove to be an awkward obstacle to further therapy. But if these barriers can be broken down, effective treatment is possible. Of course, there are occasions where this normally preliminary exercise must be re-located. It may be that it is only after an intensive investigation of the specific sexual problem has taken place that these para-sexual and extra-sexual issues may come to light.

The next stage allows some resumption of physical contact, but at this point it must not be of a sexual kind. The term 'sensate focus' is often used about this concentration on extra-genital areas. The exercises are stimulating but not directly erotic, and involve caressing of the hands, feet etc. The aim is to re-awaken the couple to the delights of their own bodies, and to create a context within which further physical experimentation will become possible. It also suggests that there are goals other than intercourse and orgasm that are important as expressions of mutual care and affection. There is a de-emphasis on performance. The couple are encouraged to concentrate on the pleasure they are deriving from these activities rather than on the activities themselves. They must try not to act as spectators of their responses or non-responses; this is not the object of the exercise. If possible they must try to take their minds off themselves and their own gratification, and concentrate on the pleasure of their partners. By indulging in a little physical altruism, they hope that their own responses will improve. But just how they control their own self-awareness so as not to look for their own responses is not really made clear. It presumably works *ex opere operato*; in the very act of sexual selflessness, the necessary expectation and confidence is generated.

Perhaps it should be added in parenthesis that, although the literature tries to make a clear distinction between marital therapy and sex therapy, the two must overlap in particular situations. In treating the symptom — whatever that may happen to be — and presumably modifying and even enhancing the patient's sexual performance, it is further assumed that his relationship(s) will also be improved. But what complicates this whole approach is the fact that, in clarifying the issues at the outset, the couple may well come to the conclusion that the only thing that they are really clear about is that they do not want to go any further with the programme. If they try the next stage of non-sexual stimulation, it may turn out to be something of a charade. There seems to be little doubt that sensate focus can be effective only where there is the predisposition to enjoy it. Caressing the extremities or whatever — with or without the use of recommended body-oils — may have a very limited function. It may help the couple to return to the old familiarity of physical contact which had to be temporarily abandoned, but it could hardly heal a fundamental rift in their relationship. Massage may be a pleasant restorative, but it can do little for a bad marriage.

Provided all has gone well, the couple can continue with the third stage of the programme. After some instruction in the techniques appropriate to their situation, the couple will then be allowed to apply these in love-play exercises that involve direct genital contacts. It is hoped that by this time some sexual self-belief will have been restored, and that these stimulatory acts will have the natural effects. Indeed, one suspects that the therapist expects that during this disciplined programme of sexual exploration the couple will exceed their brief and actually engage in intercourse. Provided there is no significant relapse, there is a sense in which — from the therapist's point of view — there can be success even in failure. This is quite likely to occur where impotence is being treated specifically.

In cases of erectile dysfunction, it is normally essential to reduce the expectations for adequate performance, and in its way this applies just as much to the partner, if available, as to the patient. Making impossible demands of the patient can only exacerbate his condition. Ridicule is death, so where possible the partner's co-operation must be enlisted. In order to relieve pressure on the patient, he has to be given a series of modified sexual goals. Some form of sensate focusing can be useful here. Actual intercourse must be seen as only one of a variety of means to sexual satisfaction. Caressing can be regarded as a minor end in itself; and certainly manual, oral or even mechanical stimulation are considered to be not only pleasurable, but equally legitimate ways of achieving orgasm. To this end, the patient may be encouraged simply to 'pleasure' his partner, to concentrate on her needs to the exclusion of his own. In doing this, he may become less preoccupied with his own fears. Consequently, the excitement he is generating in his partner may trigger his own natural responses. Alternatively, the partner may stimulate him both manually and orally. The technique here is to induce an erection which is then allowed to subside; the penis is then re-stimulated, but care is taken not to bring the man to orgasm. This may be repeated several times on any one occasion; again, not only is it pleasurable in itself, but it also 'proves' to the patient that erection can be restored.

In addition to these masturbatory exercises, the woman, having stimulated her partner to erection, may practise brief periods of partial intromission usually from a woman-superior position. Again the aim is to try to banish performance fears, and convince him that erection can be maintained. By obvious and basic operations such as these, confidence may gradually be re-established, and the patient may 'feel himself' again. Very soon, it is hoped that full and mutually satisfying intercourse will be possible.

This is the theory, but it is not always the practice. Progress is not always as smooth as this, and even where it is possible to move from stage to stage, the time intervals may be considerable. In these cases, many therapists believe that some source of further stimulus is required to accelerate the proceedings. Three kinds of possible stimulus are normally used in addition to the exercises (although these are not necessarily endorsed by Masters and Johnson themselves). They fall into fairly distinct categories, but to some extent they can be used in conjunction with one another.

First, there is the use of mechanical aids. These can range from simple pressure rings fitted to the base of the penis to 'hold' the erection, to the use of various forms of vibrator. The latter are normally associated with female masturbation, but have been used by both sexes with varying degrees of success. More eccentrically, there are the very bizarre inflatable sex dolls with which men can simulate sex play and even intercourse, but which are probably used by only a tiny minority of patients. Second, and perhaps more commonly, there is the use of fantasy combined with what are known technically — and perhaps euphemistically — as 'sexually explicit materials'. These are what most people would probably categorize as pornographic. They can be oral: records and tapes for the bedroom not infrequently consisting of whispered intimacies followed by the rising crescendo of sexual activity.

Japanese erotica seem to be currently in fashion; the sounds of sex are universal. More usually, they are visual: magazines, colour slides and films are commonly used, often as a basis for fantasy. These may consist mainly of nude figures, often in provocative poses, or they may involve scenes of actual love-making. Where it is thought necessary, explicitly 'blue' films may be used which often have an orgiastic approach to stimulation; masturbation, cunnilingus, fellatio, coitus; heterosexual, homosexual, bisexual, in every conceivable (or in this highly cautious age, non-conceivable) position, a sort of sexual Butlins — there is something for everyone.

Fantasy is an important ingredient in sex therapy. It is held that most people crave sexual experience that they never actually have, often with people that they have never actually met. For example, it is argued that women favour fantasies about sexual encounters that involve an element of force, possibly because this gives them absolution from guilt. This harks back to Freudian ideas about subliminal longings which we never really express or perhaps even acknowledge. Fantasy allows us to do this, and according to many therapists should be actively encouraged. Some therapists go so far as to insist that sexual dysfunction may be directly attributable to a poorly developed sexual fantasy life, and that it is their task to teach us how to enjoy fantasy for sexual purposes. It is regarded as a good and useful ability which can enliven the sex lives of couples whose sexual appetites have perhaps become somewhat jaded. 'People like to imagine that they are having sexual relations with new . . . people, [someone] from the entertainment world, a public figure or even royalty . . . Housewives sometimes fantasise sexual relations with frequent callers at the house: the milkman, the postman or the window cleaner' (Gillan and Gillan, 1976, p. 67). These fantasies can 'round off' chance encounters, presumably with a partner or by personal masturbation.

'Perhaps a sexual partner is not available, or a person wishes to be alone. Solitary sex can be both a necessity and a pleasure, and in either case fantasies can and should be readily conjured up as one's fancy dictates' (Gillan and Gillan, 1976, p. 67). Even more effective is the orgy or sex party. Group sex can begin, so we are told, with strip poker or games with forfeits and end up in 'a tangle of couplings or group masturbation' (Gillan and Gillan, 1976, p. 67). Failing this, for those who have neither the nerve nor the opportunity for such erotica, there is always the fantasy of sexual orgies as food for masturbation. The therapy world is a pragmatic world, so it is really all a matter of what excites you most. If it so happens, as with the impotent male, that the actualities do not come at all readily, then this retraining with sexually explicit materials is always available either as a therapeutic aid or simply, as a source of mental gratification.

What can be done if mechanical and other erotic aids are unsuccessful? They can and do provide a form of stimulus for some men, but it has no lasting effect. As Martin Cole puts it, 'pornography has a half-life of about two days'. People can become sated by pictorial sex in all its various guises; with constant exposure it can lose its effect. Some men need something more to trigger their sexual responses. Alternatively, while some men are quite capable of achieving erections fantasizing in the secrecy of their own rooms, when they actually have to perform with a partner their problems reappear. To this extent, solitary fantasies can be counter-productive; they are mere simulation exercises. When it comes to the *real* thing, it is another matter. It is for these reasons that some therapists insist that their male patients must actually be confronted with the thing they fear: a willing and active partner who is ready for intercourse. So they are prepared to supply surrogate partners for their patients as part of a treatment programme.

In probably the best-known centre for such treatment in Britain[10] the programme follows along these general lines (for further details see Cole, 1975, pp. 115ff.):

Stage 1 The social interaction stage, where the 'therapist' (surrogate)[11] helps both to relax and stimulate the patient by conversation, and by taking a keen interest on his situation.

Stage 2 The initial body contact stage, which may be reached after one or two meetings. The speed at which the programme proceeds is very much a play-it-by-ear (or whatever) process, and is usually determined by the experience and initiatives of the surrogate. In this stage mutual caressing of a non-genital kind is allowed and fantasy may be used for added erotic effect. If erection occurs it goes 'unnoticed' by the surrogate. The important feature of this stage is to avoid any kind of threatening expectations for the patient, but he can hardly be unaware of where all this is supposed to lead.

Stage 3 This is the full-body contact stage. If erection or a partial erection is obvious, clothes are removed, and caressing continues in which body creams may be used. Stimulation will be mutual. The surrogate will concentrate on the patient's pelvic region, but will try to avoid direct contact with the penis. The patient, on the other hand, may be encouraged to explore the woman's vulva, which may, for him, be a new or certainly unusual experience.

Stage 4 This genital contact stage is probably the most crucial step for the impotent male. If a sustained erection is achieved, and if it is shown that an erection can easily be re-established, then masturbation takes place either by the patient or his partner, which may or may not be to orgasm. If however failure occurs at this stage — especially when there were promising signs in Stage 3 — probably no amount of direct stimulation will work. Frantic attempts to succeed will almost certainly make the situation worse. The mental block is obviously too strong, and the surrogate must return to an earlier stage and take it from there.

Stage 5 Provided all has gone well, the patient can move to the first penetration stage. With the 'telescoping' of the normal preliminary activities, and the achievement of a firm erection, the patient is now ready for intromission. Almost invariably this is done with the surrogate adopting the woman-superior position and merely allowing the patient to enjoy intercourse without bringing him to orgasm. Needless to say, many patients do, nevertheless, ejaculate in these circumstances.

Stage 6 This is the culmination stage in which the patient, presumably having regained his sexual confidence, is ready for full intercourse. He takes the initiative, and the couple adopt any position they choose which they feel will be conducive to complete physical satisfaction.

This, again, is the theory, and in a number of cases it is also the practice. But it is a practice that does have problems. First, it is essentially a report-back system, so much depends upon the experience and reliability of the surrogates themselves. Usually, they are not prostitutes, but are volunteers — often married women — who are paid for their services. Sometimes professionals are employed,[12] but this does not necessarily ensure that they are more adept at analysing the patient's responses. It seems to be extremely rare in this country for the consultant therapist to observe surrogate therapy personally, let alone actually to engage in therapeutic sex play with the patients themselves, although therapy could be regarded as voyeurism at one remove. Therefore, they have to rely almost entirely on the reliability of the surrogate in accurately reporting back at every stage of the programme. The experience and general expertise of the surrogates is such that normally there is little need for concern, but no one is infallible.

This form of therapy can be relatively unsuccessful for a number of reasons. There are occasions when the demands of the patient are so bizarre that the surrogate feels unable to help, but it can always be argued that in these cases the patient probably had no right to be there in the first place. A more pertinent problem is where erectile dysfunction is only one manifestation of the patient's overall inadequacy, and where counselling of a more general nature is required. A third difficulty relates oddly enough to successful therapy. There is a sense in which the treatment can be too effective. The patient responds perhaps even better than anticipated, but his activities with the surrogate can be for him a kind of secondary sexual socialization. He may now be perfectly adequate with the surrogate but even more inadequate with his wife. After all, surrogates are not chosen for their physical repugnance or their frigid indifference. His wife or erstwhile regular partner may well suffer by comparison. This 'imprinting' may relate specifically to the particular surrogate who has treated him, or it may have more general applications — though not in the intended direction. In this case, there may either be a disruption of his marriage/relationship, or he will try to persevere only to find that very soon the old problems return.

It is clear from the literature that not all therapists are happy about the use of surrogates. For a variety of reasons, they will usually permit surrogate therapy only in certain cases. Masters and Johnson, who have used surrogate partners with some success, cite instances of therapists who, in effect, seduce their patients in the name of therapy. This is not, strictly, surrogate therapy as such, but it does constitute a form of 'treatment' of a surrogate nature. Their view is that there may be nothing wrong with such sex acts in themselves, but they may do little for the patient's marriage problems, and they should not be done in the guise of therapy (see Masters and Johnson, 1970, pp. 141ff.). Similar reservations are voiced by Helen Kaplan (1974, p. 227), who is the author of what is now probably the standard text on sex therapy. She criticizes those who are exploiting the current interest in sex therapy by initiating poorly conceived and sensational quasi-orgy 'therapeutic' procedures.

Success rates with these various forms of therapy from stimulation-fantasy therapy to surrogate therapy are not always easy to assess. Different figures are given by different authorities in the field, but on the whole the impression that is given is an optimistic one. Masters and Johnson make very modest claims for their success rate with primary impotent males, about 60 per cent, but with males suffering secondary impotence the figure is about 74 per cent. It has been argued that Masters and Johnson's success rates may be attributable to the highly selective nature of their clientele. In a more recent study, Bancroft (1976), using a modified form of the Masters and Johnson approach, reviewed some 200 cases which can be summarised as follows: 86 patients refused treatment or thought it inappropriate. Of the remainder:

      37% had a 'successful outcome';
      31% had 'worthwhile improvement';
      13% had 'no worthwhile improvement';
      19% dropped out.

Wolpe and Lazarus, using a variant technique, claim an 80 per cent success rate. Two further researchers, Lobitz and LoPiccolo, have found that stimulation therapy with a particular emphasis on fantasy-shaping worked with about 66 per cent of impotent men. Much the same improvement rate is given by Patricia Gillan using similar techniques. (Much of this material on success rates has been summarized by Gillan and Gillan, 1976, pp. 205-6.) In the United States, Hartman and Fithian, using films depicting intercourse, also claimed rates similar to those of Masters and Johnson; Helen Kaplan, while stating that it is quite easy to 'cure' the impotent male, insists that he does not always stay cured, and mentions a 5 per cent relapse rate (Kaplan, 1974, p. 322). These figures compare very favourably with those given by some psychoanalysts with cures in about four out of ten cases after some two years of treatment (Kaplan, 1974, p. 479).

Encouraging rates of improvement are reported where certain drugs are given intravenously to induce a sense of relaxation.[13] But the issue of drug therapy, which is a source of continuous debate in the whole field of medicine, needs considerable clarification when related to the alleviation of sexual difficulties. Perhaps drug treatment has a real future in this area, but the scope for possible abuses is virtually unlimited; it is here that the serious researcher and the charlatan occupy very similar territory. Such delights as 'Penis Heat Cream — for a stinging erection and gradual enlargement of the penis' and 'Casanova Capsules — designed to help increase the frequency of sexual climax' can be confused with drug therapy that has proven, if limited, applications.

Drugs are often used in combination with behavioural techniques, and can be conveniently classified in three main categories (see Cooper, 1978):

(1) anxiety-reducing agents;
(2) hormones;
(3) antidepressants.

Where certain depressants are used, there is always the

possibility that, while relaxing the patient, they will also reduce his sexual drive and even limit his physical responses. Hormone treatment is sometimes recommended with more suggestible patients who feel that they need some 'extra male substance'. The result of this psychological-pharmocological combination can be effective in appropriate cases where patients are convinced that they require 'rejuvenation'. Antidepressants, on the other hand, tend to be used where there is an apparent loss of libido, possibly associated with more general anxieties of a domestic, vocational or financial nature. In short, there is no miracle drug for all occasions or, indeed, for all patients. Drug therapy must be employed carefully and discriminatingly in selected cases; in these conditions it can often have significant alleviate effects.

As far as surrogate therapy is concerned, Masters and Johnson report complete success with males suffering from premature ejaculation, but only about 66 per cent success with those suffering from primary and secondary impotence. Perhaps surprisingly, Martin Cole, who relies almost exclusively on surrogate treatment, claims a modest 50 per cent improvement rate.

The general outlook for the impotent male undergoing treatment is therefore encouraging; there is a better than even chance that something can be done about his condition. But, as always, there is a cautionary note. The obvious problem underlying this research concerns the key terms themselves. What *exactly* is meant by 'success'? Is it really meaningful to say, as Helen Kaplan does, that impotence is easy to 'cure' while admitting that the cure does not always last? Is an impermanent cure, by definition, a cure at all? Similarly, it is difficult to assess accurately what is meant by more modest claims in terms of 'improvement' or even 'anxiety relief'. To be fair, it is not always easy to keep check on those who claim some improvement and who now are no longer on the 'mailing-list'. Ultimately, researchers have to make assumptions. They must hope that their patients and/or their partners are giving accurate and honest data, and that 'success' is continuing where there are no reports to the contrary.

Perhaps what sex therapy needs to be most effective is not just patient confidence but a sense of 'legitimacy'. Patients have to feel not only that it will work but also that it is 'right' or natural. The purpose, after all, of these various forms of therapy is to enhance pleasure, to facilitate feeling, establish competence; in short, to give nature a chance. But this may mean the abandonment of previous inhibitions or 'standards' that are said to impede the therapeutic process. This is done by giving even the more extreme measures, such as the use of surrogate partners, a semblance of medical authentication. And it remains a matter of dispute whether it can really enjoy this kind of professional status.

Sex therapy is a growth industry. There are now some 200 doctors belonging to the Institute of Psychosexual Medicine with possibly 400 more in training. There are about sixty psychosexual clinics, the majority of which are run by the National Health Service and provide free treatment.[14] This includes the many private clinics that are also in practice. In the United States the first Institute for the Advanced Study of Human Sexuality has been established (1976) which offers both masters and doctoral degrees in many aspects of sexuality including sexual dysfunction (see *The Times Higher Educational Supplement,* 8 September 1978).

But a question that is begged about the entire sex therapy operation is the extent to which it is really necessary. This is to dispute not the value of research, but the institutionalisation of that research in terms of the sex therapy business itself. Of course, it can be argued that the research and the treatment programmes are inseparable and that one is an extension of the other. But the conclusion is unavoidable that some exploitation of a need is really taking place. The amount of literature that the research has generated suggests that self-help alternatives are now within the reach of most impotent males. It must be possible for many patients to become their own therapists, provided they can enlist the help of sympathetic and co-operative partners.

APPENDIX

The social biography will usually concentrate on familiar areas and require the following details:[15]

(1) *History of present complaint:*
Nature of problem: Does it occur under all conditions?
                     With any partner, etc.?
Duration of the problem:
Effect of the problem: on health, marriage, partner, etc.:

(2) *Previous medical history:*
Bodily functions:

(3) *Family history:*
Relationships of parents with each other, with patient, with others:
Parental attitudes:
Relationships with siblings, other relatives etc.:

(4) *Personal history:*
Occupation: hours, quality satisfaction:
Financial situation:
Marriage: relationship, common interests, points of conflict:
Children: ages, attitudes to them:
Sexual experience: early learning, education, trauma, pre extra-marital, attitudes to same and opposite sex:
Contraception: attitudes, practices:
Anxieties, fears, attitudes, drink, smoking habits, etc.:

8. Some Conclusions

Modern man has opted for a scientific orientation towards the world. This has meant that he has abandoned the old religious determinism for a rational appreciation of his situation. But in doing this, he has, perhaps unwittingly, substituted a kind of biological determinism. Little, if anything, is god-given or god-appointed anymore; man is no longer so inclined to speak of 'acts of God' or 'accidents of history'. But what has taken their place? One all-purpose demon has gone, but many have come to take its place. When this once-satisfactory explanation was considered untenable, several comparably unsatisfactory explanations were accepted instead. The opposite of believing in something may simply be to believe in anything.

The acceptance of the scientific world-view has had a number of related implications. There has been a reaction against a crude physiologicism which implied that man was completely at the mercy of his 'nature', and that no change was likely as long as his biochemistry remained the same. Instead, there has been a tacit acceptance of man's potentiality for change. But this always carries a special caveat. The snag is that, although improvability is believed to be possible, very little is actually witnessed. The assumption is always that man's nature is somewhat better than its performance. How, then, is this to be explained?

At the macro-level, in terms of general historical development, it may be thought that man's basic problem is that he is shackled to his animal nature, and that he cannot either safely release or come to terms with his primeval appetites. Alternatively, at the micro-level, psychotherapy tends towards the experiential escape route. Something in the experience of the individual — preferably as a child — inhibits his progress. It may be the favoured traumatic incident that generates a personality defect, or it may be thought to stem from the nature of the learning process. Whatever it is, it will be regarded as *outside the present capacity of the individual to influence or control,* at least not without the aid of the relevant experts. Either way, there is a retardation of development which has sexual repercussions.

In trying to correct, or at least complement, this kind of explanation, the sociologist has stepped in with his own version of the deterministic approach. Man is not so much a victim of his nature as a victim of his social situation. The spectres of socialization and stratification are introduced, and again man is seen as lost unless he develops a sense of social awareness. This, by implication, often means class awareness, and the possibility of emancipation from the dominant bourgeois ideology — concerning sex, or anything else.

All these approaches, therefore, tend to see man at the mercy of inexorable forces. He is the victim of nature, of history, indeed of his own biography. He can find release, so it is suggested, through the enlightenment which is offered by the appropriate disciplinary gurus: psychoanalysts, psychotherapists, sociologists, etc. But do these work? We have already seen that the problem of sexual dysfunction and its attendant therapies are the subjects of considerable debate. Despite the specious arguments, very little is *certain*. The causes of impotence are largely unknown, and the theories that are held to explain it are usually unverifiable. Furthermore, the therapies that are claimed to alleviate its effects still do not enjoy any real consensus. Yet having said this, there are still grounds for optimism. Certain trends can be identified, some theories do have more cogency and are more illuminating than others, and — regardless of their theoretical underpinnings — some therapies can often be most effective in the treatment of particular forms of dysfunction.

Let us look at each of these points in turn. The question of cause is probably the most contentious issue of all, and has been aggravated by the tendency to confuse what is plausible and possible with what is thought to be 'true'.

What must be made clear at the outset is that there is no such thing as an impotent *type*. No males are classic or obvious candidates, although some do share common characteristics which may be regarded as significant. These relate particularly to background and upbringing, and relationships with parents and siblings during childhood. But there is nothing invariable in all this. To establish or identify a certain pattern of socialization does not inevitably 'mark' the child irredeemably from its early years. The exceptions are legion. The truly exceptional cases, where, say, incest has been involved, are such a tiny proportion of the whole that they can probably be discounted as far as the population in general is concerned.

It is important here to differentiate between cases and trends. Cases are, by definition, individual and particular, and are therefore within the province of the psycho-sexual specialists. Trends, on the other hand, are more general, and therefore come within the scope of the social sciences. Sociology, in particular, is concerned with those areas of human conduct that can be seen to have a patterned recurrence. Sometimes this means that its theories must be formulated at such a high level of abstraction that they are virtually meaningless for everyday applications. Sociology is primarily interested in singular incidents only in so far as they illustrate underlying trends or movements. Particular wars, particular revolutions, particular crimes, etc., all have an interest in themselves, but to the sociologist *per se* their chief attraction lies in the fact that through them he may be able to plot overall patterns of social behaviour.

This same nomothetic emphasis is seen in sociological approaches to sexual problems. All individual cases are unique; therefore, in its own way, every case is interesting. Even more than this, each has its own element of poignancy, and consequently merits concern. But important as this is, the main interest for the sociologist is the way in which each case expresses some ongoing truth about the social process. Therapists are professionally concerned to treat individual need, while other academics wish to formulate universal theories about sexual dysfunction as a social phenomenon. One task is primarily alleviative, the other is cognitive. Social scientists want to know what the presence of sexual dysfunction tells us about society in general and how this is reflected in the common perceptions of its members. This involves not only the accumulation and analysis of data, but also some appreciation of the shared sexual norms of given communities, and the ways in which these are both inculcated and transmitted.

General data on male impotence is limited; research is obviously inhibited by the very nature of the problem. It is surmised that only a very small percentage of men who experience this kind of inadequacy actually seek treatment, but certain broad statements can be made by extrapolating from known studies.[1] What emerges is that the impotent male is no *one* kind of a person. All kinds of men experience these difficulties, and only in very few specific ways do they differ significantly from the general male population.

Presenting patients tend to come from the top three social classes (on the Registrar General's classification); this reflects the general figures for the population as a whole. What may be important, however, is that some research[2] shows that the percentage of patients from

Class II is nearly double that for the population. This could be explained in a number of possible ways. It does not necessarily signify that the lower classes are more potent; it may simply mean that they too have problems but are reluctant to seek treatment. Higher-class males probably have a more sophisticated awareness of their condition, and can afford to do something about it. Possibly it also supports the pressure-of-work hypothesis; difficulties of this kind are presumably more likely to affect the professional man who is absorbed by business worries.

The mean age of presenting patients at The Institute for Sex Education and Research at Birmingham is 32.1 years, which would seem to be rather low, but it may be that this can be accounted for by the probability that fewer older men present themselves for therapy on the assumption that their condition is simply a function of age. In a resigned way, they may give themselves up as hopeless cases.

As might be expected, impotent males are not greatly in evidence among the married. They are very underrepresented in the lower-age married categories: in the 25—34 age group patients only 38 per cent are married, compared with an 80 per cent marriage rate for the general population. This changes considerably in the older categories, where in the 45—54 group the figure is 83 per cent married compared with 90 per cent for the population as a whole.[3] At the same time, it is worth noting that in presenting patients the figure for those divorced and separated is also, not surprisingly, high.

The dominant mother/father hypothesis — greatly revered by many psychotherapists — shows an interesting twist. The father appears to be the dominant parent in the case of impotent males, while the mother is the dominant parent of those experiencing premature ejaculation. What this signifies is difficult to know, but what can be said is that there is no marked evidence of homosexuality, which tends to undermine the view that men may fail in heterosexual encounters because they are really latently homosexual.

Martin Cole has found that only 54 per cent of his patients have any religious beliefs. This qualifies the companion hypothesis that many men are impotent because they are riddled with feelings of guilt deriving from the sexual proscriptions of narrow religious teachings.

Despite these ambiguities, Dr Cole's research findings are valuable, and may help indirectly in the relief of considerable suffering. One of the saddest facts to emerge is that attempted suicide among dysfunctional males is twice the national average. Impotence often either accompanies or results from forms of acute depression (see Haslam, 1978).

These are the trends, but what causes impotence in given *individual* cases is the province of the biomedical sciences. Investigations continue, and biochemistry will presumably have more to say on the subject. But in the *para*-medical field, psychotherapy may have to modify or even abandon some of its prevailing theoretical models, particularly the Freudian constructs which make little contribution to our understanding of the problem. Indeed, in concentrating its efforts on the search for hypothetical origins, however laudable, it may be neglecting the more urgent task of perfecting practical therapies to alleviate the condition. What is particularly interesting is that, while the therapies that are now being applied are largely behavioural in emphasis, there is still a tendency to fall back on the Freudian legacy for explanatory purposes. And, as we have seen, it is doubtful whether this has any scientific or even practical validity.

It is sometimes tempting to think that researchers with a penchant for physiological explanations are on the right track when they speculate about the biochemical basis of the problem. If this should prove to be the case, presumably it will only be a matter of time before impotence can be suitably treated by the appropriate drugs (see Johnson 1968). But, as yet, this is all very uncertain. Even if it is largely a biochemical matter, we still need to know how and in what circumstances it is triggered in actual cases. We know that on specific occasions the prevailing conditions produce an 'override' effect which neutralizes the normal biological drives. What exactly these conditions are, and how they operate for given individuals, cannot always be determined. Fortunately, these explanatory doubts need not necessarily reduce the effectiveness of certain therapies for certain patients. The theories and the therapies do not *have* to go together.

The importance of context is related to that of perception. Ideas about sex are among the most common 'given' elements in any society. Every individual, no matter what his cultural background, is acquainted with the traditional sexual lore and quickly develops an awareness of his own place in the socio-sexual order. Sex as a procreative activity; sex simply as pleasure; sex as something to be controlled; sex as the great liberator.[4] In a sense, man's sexual reality is already socially constructed for him (see Berger and Luckmann, 1969). For the young, especially, there is always the ideology of the super-sexual male, and what it means to be 'potent' and 'masculine' and 'virile' are just some of the received 'truths' that shape their thinking. Therefore, their personal perceptions of their own sexuality are crucially important to their development. Their feelings of superiority or inferiority, their experience or non-experience, their acceptance or non-acceptance, must all be inextricably bound up with their sense of sexual confidence or otherwise.

Male perceptions of sexual role will be largely coloured by their interactions with others whom they regard as particularly significant[5] and from whom they tend to take their sexual cues, their peer group and, not least of all, their actual or intended sexual partners. Ironically, perhaps one of the male's main problems is that he is intimidated by a reified sexual image. He may have an idealized mental construct of the kind of sexual being he would either like to be or *ought* to be, but be unable to measure up to this idealization. In an atmosphere of greater frankness about the explicit nature of the male sexual role, many men may feel incapable of meeting these demands.[6]

But how valid are these levels of expectation, and on what unambiguous bases can they possibly have been established? There are no certain data here, even the attempts that have been made to correlate performance with class position, etc., have never yielded any satisfactory conclusions (Fink, 1974). Perhaps men are largely at the mercy of their own sexual mythology. Any kind of implicit performance ethic must be treated with caution.[7] Consequently, the emphasis on sex as simply technique must similarly be abjured. The assumption in so many of the sex manuals, that performance can be faultless if the rules are faithfully followed, is misconceived. There are probably too many stereotypes as to what women are supposed to want of men in love-making (de Martino, 1974, pp. 271-2). But such ideas are very hard to undermine. It is interesting that Ann Welbourne, after handling 15,000 telephone questions at the Community Sex Information Centre, New York City, found that eight out of ten men — mostly single and in their twenties — asked mainly about the mechanics of sex. The error is that technique is mistaken for knowledge (see the discussion in Nichols, 1975). Sex is not merely a series of structured responses, and human relationships are more than a complex of fixed roles.

Perhaps, therefore, one of the most significant factors in male sexual dysfunction is the change that is said to be taking place in the perceptions of his sexual role. This involves not only the much-vaunted assertion of female sexuality, but also what is regarded as the rediscovery of a natural bisexual order, and the consequent emphasis on the possible interchangeability of sexual roles. The suggestion is that, with increasing differentiation in society and the subsequent variability of social tasks, there has arisen a need for a realignment of sexual roles. In effect, this has meant that men particularly have had to adapt to a new socio-sexual situation in which their prerogatives have been increasingly usurped by women. By way of compensation, however, they have been given more latitude in the area of homosexual relations. But as this has also been extended to women, it could be argued that, on balance, men have lost out in the sexual stakes. Thus, the male sexual role is now said to be unclear, and this in turn is thought partly to account for the increasing incidence of dysfunctionality. In short, the implication is that impotence is a function of changing social roles in general, and the uncertainties of the male sexual role in particular.

However, this study maintains that this analysis is essentially mistaken. Of course, there are changing perceptions of sexual roles, although it is doubtful whether they can be called 'new'. There is little that is sexually new under the sun. Even the indirect control of fertility, normally associated with the scientific age, was anticipated in many ancient societies which practised institutionalized abortion and infanticide. It is true that both men and women are adapting to a changing situation, but their basic sexual roles have not really altered. There is nothing really opaque about the traditions of sexual practice. Men *know* what is expected of them. It is not so much uncertainty as *certainty* of role that troubles them. There may, of course, be doubtful role delineations. Specificities of sexual role relate to the perennial problem of the institutionalization of sexual practice. When procedures are informal and 'understood' there are often fewer difficulties than when attempts are made to define and standardize them.

We live in times when the image of super-sexuality has taken institutionalized forms. Directly and indirectly, sexual athleticism is being promoted, especially by the media, and this gives it the gloss of respectability. What was once private has become public; what was confined to rumour and innuendo is now committed to print and media portrayal. It is a plausible hypothesis that the modern mechanization of sex has led to the creation of artificial performance levels. As we have seen, some men may feel that they cannot compete, and this has resulted in a higher incidence of sexual inhibition and even dysfunction. This competitive approach to sex necessarily involves a continual checking of one's own performance levels, perhaps against the supposed standards of others. Deliberation of this kind can spell doom to actual sexual action. One of the strange inconsistencies of society is that, while so many of its norms are related to what is known to be possible, some norms are elevated to the rank of *ideals* and then achievement always falls short of intention. Striving is always a noble aim, but perhaps some men just expect too much of themselves.

Most responses to difficult situations are either of a flight or fight variety. To retreat can be ultimately catastrophic. It leads, in some cases, to an eventual paralysis of the will. But where the decision is made to fight a problem, this determination must be accompanied by sincere self-examination. Self-doubt can so easily lead to self-deception, which is then disguised by excuses and rationalizations. In sexual situations self-honesty may necessarily involve admissions to partners which they might find difficult to accept. But this may be the essential pre-condition for rebuilding a person's self-image and restoring his self-esteem.

Having said this, however, it would be a mistake for men to confuse knowing themselves and their own limitations with an obsessively reflexive attitude towards their own sexuality. *Self*-knowledge is not the same as having *sexual* knowledge. Of course, it is useful to be acquainted with the techniques, and to be aware of the physiological and psychological facts. But when this results in an extreme sensitivity about performance it can be disastrous. Both the technical and practical knowledge of sex are necessary, but the kind of hyper-intellectuality that is all too conscious of everything that can go wrong is fatal. Perhaps this is one of the great disadvantages of the 'new' openness about sex, and with it the seemingly inexhaustible production of treatises on sex research. We can perhaps know *too* much about the problems. Knowledge of this sort can be an encumbrance. Ignorance was not necessarily bliss, but there is more than a germ of truth in the old allegation that we did not have sexual neuroses until the experts told us so. We are now faced with the Adam-and-Eve dilemma: if we insist on eating of the Tree of Knowledge, we must be prepared to face the responsibilities that it brings.

For men, therefore, to be forever preoccupied with their own capacities and incapacities can have crippling effects on their sexual activity (see Nichols, 1975, pp. 205ff.). But how can this possibly be avoided? For a person to say to himself 'while I am doing this, I must never think of *that*' is merely to remind himself of the awful possibilities. It is clearly a negative reinforcement of the fear. He would like to be able to relax, to take things as they come, but he finds this difficult. On the other hand, if he tries to 'fight' his impotence, he feels that he is simply reminding himself of its very futility. Saying 'I *will* go to sleep' merely tends to prolong insomnia. Yet perhaps he should respond to his condition more aggressively: not to withdraw, not to disengage, not to shy away from opportunities to 'prove' himself, but instead to face the problem head-on regardless of the disappointments and the sense of frustration.

Fear, then, is really the key problem. And this means

fear at several levels. At the most general level, as we have seen, fear can be generated by an imaginative projection of all the worst possibilities (rather like reading a medical dictionary and suspecting that all one's symptoms indicate something quite mortal). More specifically, fear can be precipitated by just one 'natural' failure which cannot be overlooked by either partner. This may be occasioned by something quite simple — tiredness, financial difficulties, business worries or some form of domestic tension. None of these things is directly related to sex, but the sex *act* may be attempted when the male is sub-consciously preoccupied with a problem of this kind. As far as research can ascertain, failure in these or similar circumstances is not at all uncommon, and should — as far as is possible — be disregarded by both partners. The man should not be thought of as some sort of oddity. Failure of this kind should be seen as a temporary aberration which may rarely, if ever, be repeated. It cannot be stressed enough that failure in these conditions is not fatal, even if the man is unable to adduce any obvious, or even not so obvious reasons for it. This is something he is bound to do, but he should not let this destroy his sexual confidence or inhibit love-making on a future occasion. If he does, he is likely to enter a fear syndrome in which each unsuccessful attempt becomes the cause of subsequent failure. So what began as a particular cause producing a particular effect will have developed into a situation in which a specific effect has become a general cause.

Because of the traumatic nature of failure, some men find it very difficult to adopt a reasoning attitude to their problem. The 'original' failure may have to be looked at in multi-variable terms; that is to say, there may be a complex of perhaps quite trivial reasons for it which they find too tortuous to disentangle. But whether there are many reasons or just one, there *has* to be a cause. There *is* a reason, and almost certainly it will not be necessary to dredge the unconscious mind for hidden Freudian possibilities. Not all men have a fear of the vagina because it symbolizes a demanding mother, or have poor erections because of a hypothesized competition with their fathers.[8] Failure should not, therefore, be regarded as something mysterious from which one suffers. The roots of the problem must, in theory, be discernible. Nothing is *un*caused. It is one thing to be deterministic, but quite another to be fatalistic.

Some men prefer flight, and investigators have argued that the reasons that patients give for their evasion of sexual activity are often suspect. Perhaps they have had one or more failures, and anticipate further trouble, so they try to avoid added humiliation by excuses of one kind or another. References to domestic or business responsibilities, or even age, researchers say, can be regarded as variants of the 'fatigue' argument, while allusions to moral scruples may simply indicate that the individual is afraid of women. It is suggested that some men insist on thinking of their impotence as 'penis failure' rather than failure of what is referred to as the 'whole man'. Their studies show that some men who are sexually impotent are also 'impotent' in other respects, particularly in their work situations (Milne and Hardy, 1976, pp. 108ff.).

All this, of course, begs the proverbial chicken-and-egg question. Do men with business worries carry them to bed, or does depression about failure affect their commercial judgements? It also tends to discount the possibility that there *is* no disguise, that 'excuses' really *are* reasons. More importantly, to speak of impotent men in this generalized sense suggests an impotent personality, someone who is ineffectual in many if not most of his activities. This is a highly debatable concept for which proof is singularly lacking. It, therefore, needs to be reiterated that every failure has its cause or causes; if there is a reason for it then it must be amenable to investigation and presumably to treatment.

As we have already seen, it is sometimes argued that fears of this kind may be enhanced by the heightened sexual expectations of women. Masters and Johnson, in a salutary reversal of the liberation ethic, insist that it is women who must be unchauvinistic and learn not to treat men as sex-objects. Either way, this theme has been a little overplayed. Perhaps sex can never be basically anything other than achievement-oriented. The self-giving, mutual-satisfaction approach of many sexologists must involve a giving-to-get operation; giving something successfully, in this case the partner's orgasm, results in personal gratification. No matter how altruistic its guise, sex is essentially hedonistic.

For many men, there is a kind of languid habituation about love-making. Excitement can actually be neutralized by regularity and predictability. Familiarity — the same times, the same place — can be reassuring, but it also has its disadvantages. No one is suggesting irregular excursions to the greenhouse or a mackintosh in the park, but sexual anxiety might be reduced if there was more emphasis on variety and spontaneity. Particularly important may be the shift from intercourse as an exclusive goal to other forms of pleasuring activity. Performance pressure might actually be more effectively canalized if there was greater operational altruism, with *more* — rather than less — concentration on the needs of the female partner. This tends to give the male *increased* control in a sexual situation.

Self-recognition, then, does not mean self-resignation. The kind of conversion therapy used for drug addicts and alcoholics is not necessarily recommended for those suffering from sexual failure. It is not essential for the male who is undergoing a dysfunctional phase simply to give up and 'declare' that he is impotent. His situation is quite different from that of the person who acknowledges that he is an alcoholic even though, at the present time, he may not take a drink. Definitionally, there cannot be an impotent man who, at the present time, is having regular intercourse. Labelling does not *have* to be a problem for the secondarily impotent male. Given all the qualifications that can be made about the nature and forms of sexual dysfunction, he does not have to consider himself branded indelibly as impotent. His real problem is *self*-labelling; it is not how other people regard him, but what he thinks of himself that will largely determine how he reacts to his situation (see the discussion by Plummer, 1976, albeit in a different context). This refusal to recognize that dysfunction is the norm will probably work better for most individuals. After all, their condition is almost certainly only partial and temporary, so the more they are convinced of their own basic normality, the better.

The position of the impotent male has been aggravated by the aretification of sex, that is to say, the situation where natural capacities have become elevated to the rank of psycho-social 'virtues'. What should be very nearly as natural as breathing has become that which one is 'good at'. A complimentary sexual performance becomes rather like praise for eating well. It is a false value, and an undue preoccupation with proficiency levels can be a damaging exercise. This is not to suggest that the 'natural man' is the possessor of an uninhibited sexuality, and that if we could simply strip away the veneer of socialization all would be well. Nor is it a way of applauding the capacities of the non-intellectualized man; the modern sexual primitive can also have his problems. What *is* being said is that sex is something we can all do — it needs no special talents. Some people may have sexual difficulties; they may have aberrations; but whatever they have it is probably neither unique nor particularly unusual.[9] And in most cases, it is susceptible to some form of therapy.

If there is an essential naturalness about sexuality, it follows that its expression can be enhanced. How then does the impotent male attack his problem? Can he possibly break the cycle? If he once becomes convinced that his condition is not chronic, and refuses to accept it as the norm, recovery has already begun. In some cases, a reduction of performance pressure can be helpful, especially where the male is going through the initial re-orientation stage. Much, perhaps most, current sex therapy is concerned with the minimization of anxiety, and various techniques are employed to try to achieve this. Therapeutic strategies range from history-taking and 'self-disclosure' procedures to de-sensitization techniques, and then on to written and monitored exercises, depending upon the specific nature of the problem (see for example McCarthy, 1977). These can be useful, particularly where couples are being treated together, but it may not be so effective for the male alone. His is rather a special, but not uncommon, case. An underlying difficulty with these approaches is that they can perpetuate many of the problems they set out to solve. They tend to confirm fears of inadequacy by drawing attention to the complexities of the condition that they are designed to treat. By a series of programmed rituals they may reinforce rather than reduce the levels of anxiety.

What may be more stimulating, in some cases, is for the male to *accept* or even *create* challenging situations and actually raise his sexual expectations. Of course, he will have to pace himself, and initially be content with the achievement of secondary sexual goals, but even so this constitutes an active engagement rather than a retreat from the problem. Many behaviourists might argue that this could involve the use of excitatory aids and the adoption of innovatory techniques. The difficulty is that improvisation patterns can be established — as in jazz — so that each act of creativity becomes limited and even stereotyped. The behavioural *sine qua non* is that, given sufficient stimulation, there will be the necessary response.

This may require some re-education. The responses may need a brief refresher course in order to restore confidence, but given biochemical normality, if the stimulus is appropriate the body will react accordingly. And once a real break-through has taken place, and erection and intercourse successfully experienced, things should begin to go well from then on.

Retreat is easy for the impotent male. He knows that only if he tries and fails, is he to be regarded as impotent — so why try? Presumably, his attempts will be dictated on any one occasion by partner expectation, social convention or situational opportunity. But is there adequate stimulation? Logically, erectile failure must either be due to a waning or impaired sexual capacity, or result from the lack of adequate stimulus or possibly some form of negative stimulus. Given that in the vast majority of cases it is a stimulus problem, some behaviourists would contend that some quite radical re-orientation is called for. There may actually be considerable boredom with the domestic situation and what are felt to be stereotyped patterns of expectation. So would things change if new sexual partners were engaged? After all, why maintain a Morris Minor when a Jensen may be available?

Men sometimes tire of the usual sexual outlets. They want a change, even if this change exists only in their imaginations. Surely this partly accounts for the flourishing market in soft pornography. This helps men to indulge their sexual fantasies where there is neither the opportunity nor the initiative to actualize them. Fornication at one remove is safe and painless with little self-reproach and no humiliation. But what conditions the desire? To what extent, is modern man influenced by *Playboy*-type standards of beauty and sexual desirability? The open display of such 'possibilities' has really become accessible only in recent years. Is he programmed by commercial interest or do these idealized conceptions really correspond with his innate drives? Perhaps they are not really separable. If these provocative images represent his real desires, then his cravings for the *cordon bleu* delicacies may mean that the simple domestic fare suffers by comparison.

Impotence can be occasioned by apprehension, and this can be related, as we have seen, to all manner of causes. But in many cases it may well derive from an essential lack of desire. Sex may be a biological drive, but it is not an appetite like the need for food and drink. People can live without sex, and many do, without any visible ill-effects or neuroses. Despite the strength of the sexual urge, it is subject to various cultural imperatives. This is, of course, also true of other appetitional factors. Biologically, all humans need to eat, but *what* they eat, and particularly *how* they eat and *who* they eat with, express socially induced responses. Similarly with sex. Appetites are not insatiable, and it should not be assumed that everyone has a limitless reservoir of sexuality which is just waiting to be released, or that this release can always be triggered in the same way in every individual. Even animals often need the right conditions in which to mate, and — on the most cynical estimate — men are not exactly animals. The civilizing process, for good or ill, has endowed them with certain sensitivities about sex which must condition its expression. The female can mate without any urgent wish to do so; desire will enhance the experience, but it is not a necessary pre-condition of the act. This is not normally the case with the male. He either wants or he does not want. Rarely can this be conjured up to order. It cannot be generated artificially. His erectile response will then normally be a function of his desire, and this in turn will be triggered by the appropriate stimuli. These cannot be duty or habit, but must be specifically erotic. A man may not want if he does not feel himself to be wanted in return. Reciprocation of desire will certainly help, but may not be essential. What *is* essential is that, in a sexual situation, the male has got to find his partner exciting if he is going to be excited himself. If he does not, nothing is going to make him. Of course, a responsive partner does not always guarantee success; prostitutes can be attractive, but they may not generate sexual anticipation. Similarly, an established partner may give reassurance, while a new partner may arouse ambivalent feelings of excitement and apprehension. For many men, the cultural override is more powerful than the physical cues.

Whether a man adopts an aggressive or a retreatist approach to the problem will depend very much upon courage, opportunity and his sense of priorities. But nothing is guaranteed. Even with the application of professional therapy or attempts at self-therapy, failure can still occur, and may only be overcome with patience and determination. But no therapy is a substitute for really *wanting,* and no technique can make up for desire. As Teilhard de Chardin once put it, 'At what moment do lovers come into the most complete possession of themselves if not when they are lost in each other?'

A process of re-education and re-habituation then may be necessary for the restoration of sexual confidence. But *understanding* is better than knowing, and the modern behavioural concentration on the symptom rather than the cause, valuable as this can be, may leave the patient in doubt as to the ostensible permanence of his cure. Understanding the reasons, which may not be that elusive, is the most essential part of any therapy. Indeed, perhaps the modern crisis of potency itself is essentially a crisis of meaning.

Notes

CHAPTER 1

1. Kinsey lists 66 reported cases out of his sample of 4,108 respondents. This included only 6 cases in those (1,627) men under twenty-five.
2. The male orgasmic 'process' is very similar. See Masters and Johnson (1966).
3. There are cases where men may be sexually excited and ejaculate with a flacid penis, but as far as can be ascertained, such cases are rare. See Kaplan (1974, p. 256).
4. Complementarily, in *legal* terms impotence is the inability of either party to consummate the marriage, i.e. for the penis to penetrate the vagina, and constitutes grounds for a possible annulment.
5. Note the discussion in Katchadouriann and Lunde (1972, pp. 306-7).
6. Some reservations concerning the general conclusions of Masters and Johnson on the matter of differential response patterns should be noted. (1966, pp. 107-10).
7. See Katchadourian and Lunde (1972, chapter 3) for an excellent summary, but which also includes the arguable assertion that orgasm can probably be experienced at all ages.
8. In the wake of new physiological data, there has been a shift away from the dual-orgasm hypothesis by the psychologists. See for example, Salzman (1968, pp. 123-45).
9. For example, Koedt (1970).
10. For a very able criticism of the emancipated by the emancipated, see Greer (1971).
11. In some ways this is analagous to the male experience. The tactile stimulation of the glans and shaft of the penis trigger the orgasm which is expressed by rhythmic reflex muscle contractions at the base of the penis.
12. J. Olds (1956) has carried out animal studies which show that erection and ejaculation can be independent of each other.
13. In their valuable text Katchadourian and Lunde (1972) refer to vasocongestion and myotonia as mechanisms that 'explain' how various sex organs respond to stimulation (p. 62). It is a common mistake,

which is made particularly by social scientists, to think that something is being explained when in fact it is only being *described*.
14. It is important to note that even a man who is unconscious or who has had an injury to his spinal cord which prevents impulses reaching the brain may still be capable of an erection given the appropriate genital stimulation.
15. See, for example, Nefzawi, *The Perfumed Garden* (trans. R. Burton) London, Neville Spearman, 1963. edn
16. Expanding this analogy, it might be argued that after the discarding of the ovum at menstruation, the time taken in uterine preparation for the possibility of fertilization constitutes the woman's reproductive 'refractory period'.
17. *Coitus reservatus* was cultivated as a sexual technique particularly in India, and was also practised by the Oneida religious community in New York State in the nineteenth century.

CHAPTER 2

1. The mean is what is normally regarded as an average i.e. taking the measurement or numerical factor for each member and dividing the total by the number of members. But there are other ways of computing an average: by taking the midpoint, or *median,* in a linear series, or by identifying the most frequently occurring measurement, the *mode.*
2. For a critique of the Kinsey studies in particular, see Lieberman (1971).
3. After his successful encounter with the prophets of Baal on Mount Carmel, we are informed (1 Kings, 19) that the prophet Elijah, in fear and uncertainty, fled to a cave convinced of the singularity of his own situation. It was there that the 'revelation' came that he and his problem were not unique.
4. This use of the term 'rationality' is customarily associated with the writer, Max Weber; see his *Theory of Social and Economic Action* (1964).
5. Note especially the attitudes of a number of Bantu societies on the matter of illegitimacy; see Fox (1967).
6. In the Ford and Beach study (1951) about one-third of the societies investigated disapproved of homosexual behaviour.
7. Among the limited number of studies, see particularly Rubin (1965).
8. The 55–69 age group sample consisted of only 51 patients, and the 70-and-over sample, 50 patients. See Finkle *et al.* (1959).
9. Studies at Duke University by Eric Pfeiffer reported in an article, 'Sex and Aging' Pfeiffer, (1975).
10. Testosterone is the only hormone secreted by the testes, the male sexual glands. It is partially responsible for sexual development in a

male direction. Androgens, a more general term, includes testosterone, adrenal and other hormones that have a virilizing testosterone-like action.
11. There are some hopes for amyl-nitrate, which increases vascular response, and for neurotransmitters such a L-Dopa, which is currently used in the treatment of Parkinson's disease, but its side-effects can sometimes be rather disturbing.
12. The much-quoted line is from Shakespeare's Macbeth (Act II Scene 3 line 34): '[Drink] provokes the desire, but it takes away the performance'.
13. Euthemic, from the Greek 'euthemeia' = desire (of the eyes) or perhaps, better still, lust.
14. Anti-cholinergic drugs act on the parasympathetic nerves, and may well be used in the treatment of peptic ulcers, and even opthalmic disorders such as iritis and glaucoma.
15. See the very useful tables in Kaplan (1974, p. 102).
16. Erich Goode (1974) quotes Dr Thaddeus Mann, Professor of Physiology of Reproduction at Cambridge University: 'Drugs serve as a sex substitute . . . [their use] . . . stems from decreased capability and is a pathetic attempt at overcoming . . . sexual incompetence'.
17. Obviously, the majorities vary with the studies in question. For a summary, see Goode (1974).

CHAPTER 3

1. The Laws of Manu. For a valuable summary, see Meyer (1953).
2. For example, the Mesopotamian myths relating to Enki and Ninhursag. For a summary, see Kirk (1976, pp. 90ff.).
3. See the Greek myths of Pasiphae and the bull or Leda and the Swan. Graves (1966).
4. Compare the various sexual exploits of, say, the Olympian Zeus or the Hindu god, Krishna who was reputed to have 16,000 wives.
5. For cursory discussions of these themes, see Bullough (1976).
6. Aristophanes. *Amphiareus* — of which only fragments are extant — tells how an old man takes his young bride on a pilgrimage in the hope of restoring his youthful vigour.
7. Onions are listed with mussels, crabs, snails and eggs as stimulants: Alexis, quoted by Licht (1932, p. 513).
8. Vatsyayana, among his detailed instructions for mutual sexual enjoyment, lists, for example — with minor variations — eighty-four different positions for intercourse: Vatsyayana, *Kama Sutra,* trans. Richard Burton, New York, Dutton (1962. edn).
9. Some sects such as the Lingayats (phallus worship) and Saktas (vagina worship) were wholly committed to a religious sexual orientation: see Meyer (1953).

10. See Bullough (1976, p. 260). This is a very useful and comprehensive general text on sexual practice.
11. 'But one must also know the art of sexual intercourse to achieve . . . extra years. If ignorance of the sexual art causes frequent losses of sperm to occur, it will be difficult to have sufficient energy . . . ': Quoted by James Ware (1966, p. 105)
12. For example, among Muslims there were several types of eunuch, depending on the exact nature of the operation involved. Where the testicles only were removed, erection was sometimes possible, but the most highly prized were those who had had the penis amputated as well (the 'tailless ones'): these were rare however because the mortality rate after the operation was so high (Bullough, 1976, p. 232).

CHAPTER 4

1. For instance, the *Journal of Sex Research*. From time to time the papers of various symposia are also published as specialized Readers.
2. For example, see the series of popular articles on the 'Sexperts' in the *Sunday Mirror* from 2 January 1977, which concentrate on problems and therapies.
3. Anita Blum, a London Marriage Guidance counsellor.
4. Note, for example, the insistence of Dr A. Wakeling, a consultant psychiatrist at the Royal Free Hospital, London, that 'there is no norm as such . . . Sexual capacity varies as much as height and weight.'
5. Professor Giovanni Caletti, commenting on the sexual behaviour of Italians.
6. Attributed to Omar Sharif, whom his reporters describe as being from the 'world of entertainment which is over-populated by two-dimensional sexists'. Perhaps it is notable that Sharif takes the view that this decline in male sexuality derives from male capitulation, and his remedy is that men must act chauvinistically — in bed, at least (Bowskill and Linacre, 1977).
7. Dr Dennis Friedman, head of the psycho-sexual dysfunction clinic at St Bartholomews Hospital, London, in an article, '45 is a Dangerous Age' *Daily Express* (28 October 1976).
8. Hodson, 1977). One would ideally wish to know rather more about the bases for some of this report's conclusions; 3,457 respondents seems high for this national but still somewhat esoteric magazine and must represent a significant proportion of the readership. Of course, it could be argued that publications of this kind have a particular appeal for the sexually uncertain, and that its readership is therefore atypical of the population as a whole.
9. Quoted in correspondence with Anna Raeburn of *Woman* magazine.
10. Reported in conversation with Dr Cole in April 1978.
11. The research has involved contacting all the main, i.e. national,

newspapers and magazines. These have been very co-operative, and have sent a wealth of cuttings, etc., which support either the general thesis of increasing incidence or increasing reportage of possible incidence.

CHAPTER 5

1. The reader might like to compare a now somewhat dated American text with similar orientations, which concentrates on correlative factors, e.g. homosexuality and impotence, alcohol and impotence, narcotics and impotence etc., which is marred by the dramatized reconstruction approach: Glover (1963).
2. Technically, a Don Juan complex should probably indicate a pervasive desire to deflower virgins, and perhaps suggests a fear of experienced women.
3. Note Case A concerning the paraphiliac in chapter 2.

CHAPTER 6

1. For an interesting discussion of these issues in the social sciences generally, see Rudner (1966).
2. One would wish to know more about these reports, but they do derive from the findings of what appears to be a reputable investigation by the *Forum* organization.
3. As a personal note, I was prescribed 'beta-blocking' drugs for migraine by a consultant neurologist. Because I was working on this project, I recognized the name, and only when I *asked* was I told that this medication could occasion erectile problems. Needless to say, I refused the drugs. Regardless of ethnomethodological theory, one can take this business of identifying with the problem too far.
4. Note the emphasis put upon the therapeutic functions of fantasy by some practitioners. See Gillan and Gillan (1976).
5. It is now reasonably well attested that tight nylon underwear cannot cope 'naturally' with the body's perspiration. The crotch particularly is 'unventilated' and becomes hot and sticky, and in these conditions the natural fungoidal balance is upset, and certain infections flourish. Although more common in the female, the male can also be affected.
6. For those with a non-Services background, the quotation should be given in full. Our hypothetical client when admonished by the possibilities of VD says, 'I don't care if I do go blind' — but always added responsibly, 'I can always sell matches.'
7. Functionalism as a theory is essentially relativist in orientation. It

follows, by definition, that if societies are functioning wholes it does violence to them to introduce alien institutions and practices that they did not generate themselves.
8. Health Education Conference, York, 11 November 1977.
9. Anthony Storr argues that reincarnatory recall is really based on cryptomnesia, that is, a fantasy based on subconscious recollections of past reading, learning, etc.
10. For a neat summary of the psychoanalytical position, see Coltart and Williams (1975).
11. Note Sigmund Freud's famous paper, *'Character and Anal Eroticism'* (1908), in which he discusses a variety of obsessional conditions relating to the anal phase.
12. It is interesting to compare the incidence of certain socially disapproved practices in the East, e.g. the increasing scale of alcoholism in the Soviet Union, which the government is making some attempts to control.
13. For a thoroughgoing examination of this interactionist approach applied to the question of male homosexuality, see Plummer (1975).

CHAPTER 7

1. The work of Masters and Johnson is very ably, if uncritically, summarized by Belliveau and Richter, (1971).
2. Female satisfaction may not even be thought desirable in some societies. It has been hypothesized that the primary reason for the practice of cliterodectomy (female circumcision) was to reduce desire in the female and presumably ensure greater fidelity.
3. For an excellent review of therapies generally, see Kovel (1978).
4. This is particularly associated with the work of J. Wolpe (1958) and H.J. Eysenck (1960).
5. Masters and Johnson's own programme normally requires that the couple live in a hotel near the clinic in St Louis for about two weeks at their own expense. This enables them to report for daily treatment while, at the same time, giving them a 'neutral' environment.
6. There is a modified — almost eclectic — form of brief psychotherapy which is still widely used in the UK. This is known as Balint therapy, and is sometimes used by doctors in general practice as a diagnostic device for trying to ascertain the 'real' nature of the patient's problem. It can be combined with genital exploration-cum-fantasy evocation techniques, and is said to have been particularly successful in the treatment of female sexual dysfunction. See Taylor (1978).
7. '... there is no such thing as an uninvolved partner in any marriage in which there is some form of sexual inadequacy': Masters and Johnson (1966).
8. The book by Helen Singer Kaplan (1974) is probably the best general book available on sex therapy, but on basic cognitive issues the author

often falls back on the unverifiabilities of neo-Freudianism.
9. In the UK, even private consultations are not likely to be as costly as in the United States. It is noteworthy that as far back as the 1960's, in their early era, Masters and Johnson were charging a full fee of $2,500 for a two-week programme exclusive of other costs — though, to be fair, not all patients were required to pay the full amount.
10. This is the Institute for Sex Education and Research at Birmingham run by Dr Martin Cole.
11. Martin Cole (1975), uses the term 'therapist' for the surrogate, presumably because she is acting therapeutically on behalf of *the* therapist, who is not actually present after the initial interviews.
12. Martin Cole, who probably uses the surrogate method more than anyone else in the UK, has about twenty or so women whom he can call upon for surrogate services. Sometimes the demands of his extensive male clientele are such that he has to enlist the co-operation of the local sauna/massage agency to augment the supply.
13. Particularly sodium amytal.
14. For an excellent summary of services available in sex therapy, see Taylor (1978).
15. This is based on an outline supplied by a GP who is also interested in sexual problems. See Strube (1975, p. 23).

CHAPTER 8

1. Some of the most valuable data available at the present time derive from the work being carried out by Martin Cole at the Institute for Sex Education and Research at Birmingham, and I am particularly indebted in this section for Dr Cole's cooperation.
2. These figures relate to Dr Cole's Institute.
3. The general population figures are taken from *Social Trends* London, HMSO, 1975.
4. For an interesting summary of the theoretical approaches that these ideas reflect, see Plummer (1975, pp. 5-8).
5. This theoretical orientation, known technically as symbolic interactionism, is particularly associated with the work of G.H. Mead, notably *The Mind, Self and Society* (1934).
6. It is all very reminiscent of the old problem of inhibitions arising from unfavourable comparisons of penis size; see Hitsch (1957, pp. 49-52).
7. Note that this sentiment is echoed even by some who might be thought to represent the liberated woman; see Greer (1972).
8. This kind of causal connection has been seriously hypothesized; see Milne and Hardy (1976, pp. 108ff.).
9. 'Most men won't ask other men, nor would they be likely to get a straight answer if they did; the level of lying in sexual matters is very early raised to the incorrigible. Hence each man thinks that his failure is in some way exceptional.' Sheehy (1976, pp. 442-3).

Bibliography

ABSE, D. WILFRED (1974) 'Sexual disorder and marriage' in D.W. ABSE et al. *Marital and Sexual Counselling in Medical Practice* New York, Harper & Row.

BANCROFT, J. (1976) 'Three years' experience of a sexual problems clinic' *British Medical Journal,* 26 June.

BARTELL, GILBERT (1971) 'Group sex among the mid-Americans' in B. LIEBERMAN (ed.) *Human Sexual Behaviour* New York, John Wiley.

BEACH, FRANK (1966) 'Review of human sexual response' *Scientific American* vol. 216, no. 2.

BEAUMONT, G (1974) 'Sexual side-effects of drugs' *British Journal of Sexual Medicine* vol. 1, no. 5, pp. 10-12.

BEAUMONT, G (1976) 'Untoward effects of drugs on sexuality' in S. CROWN (ed.) *Psychosexual Problems* pp. 333-4, New York, Academic Press.

BECKER, P. (1958) *Shaka Zulu* St Albans, Panther.

BELLIVEAU, FRED and RICHTER, LIN (1971) *Understanding Human Sexual Inadequacy* New York, Coronet Books.

BERGER, P. and LUCKMANN, T. (1969) *The Social Construction of Reality* Harmondsworth, Penguin.

BIGGS, ROBERT (1967) Ancient Mesopotamian potency incantations in texts from cuneiform sources II

BOWSKILL, D. and LINACRE, A. (1977A) *Men: the Sensitive Sex* London, Muller.

BOWSKILL, D. and LINACRE, A. (1977B) 'Virility: is it a major casualty of the sex war? *Over 21* June.

BRECHER, EDWARD (1972) *The Sex Researchers* St Albans, Panther.

BRYANT, A.T. (1949) *The Zulu* Natal South Africa, Shuter & Shooter.

BULLOUGH, VERN (1976) *Sexual Variance in Society and History* New York, John Wiley.

BURTON, R. (trans.) (1934) *A Thousand and One Nights* Heritage Press.

CARLTON, ERIC (1973) *Patterns of Belief* London, Allen & Unwin.

CARLTON, ERIC (1977) *Ideology and Social Order* London, Routledge & Kegan Paul.
CARR, JEAN (1977) 'Sexperts' *Sunday Mirror* 2 January.
CAUTHERY, PHILIP (1975) 'Man at bay' *Sunday Times* 26 October.
CAUTHERY, PHILIP and COLE, MARTIN (1971) *The Fundamentals of Sex* London, W.H. Allen.
COCHRAN, W. *et al.* (1953) 'Statistical problems of the Kinsey Report' *Journal of the American Statistical Association* vol. 48 no. 264, December, pp. 673-716.
COLE, MARTIN (1975) 'Human sex behaviour and sex therapy' in S. JACOBSON (ed.) *Sexual Problems* London, Elek.
COLSON, E. (1951) 'The Plateau Tonga of Northern Rhodesia' in E. COLSON and M. GLUCKMAN (eds) *Seven Tribes of British Central Africa* Oxford, Oxford University Press.
COLTART, NINA and WILLIAMS, A. HYATT (1975) 'The psychology of sexual development' in S. JACOBSON (ed.) *Sexual Problems* London, Elek.
CONTENAU, G. (1969) *Everyday Life in Babylon and Assyria* London, Edward Arnold.
COOPER, A. *et al.* (1970) British Medical Journal 3/17.
COOPER, A. (1978) 'Drugs in the treatment of sexual inadequacy' *British Journal of Sexual Medicine* vol. 5, April/May.
COOPER, WENDY (1976) 'Men muscle in on the menopause' *Sunday Times* 10 October.

DE JOUVENEL, B. (1963) *The Art of Conjecture* London, Weidenfeld & Nicolson.
DE MARTINO, M. (1974) 'Mistakes men make in lovemaking' in L. GROSS (ed.) *Sexual Behaviour* Flushing New York, Spectrum.
DEVEREUX, G. (1937) *Institutionalized Homosexuality of the Mohave Indians* Detroit, Wayne State University Press.

EYSENCK, H.J. (1960) *Behaviour Therapy and the Neuroses* London, Pergamon.
EYSENCK, H.J. and WILSON, G.D. (1973) *The Experimental Study of Freudian Theories* London, Methuen.

FINK, PAUL (1974) 'Duration of intercourse' in L. GROSS (ed.) *Sexual Behaviour* Flushing New York, Spectrum.
FINKLE, A. *et al.* (1959) 'Sexual potency in ageing males' *Journal of the American Medical Association* vol. 170, pp. 1391-3.
FLACELIERE, ROBERT (1973) *Love in Ancient Greece* Westport Connecticut, Greenwood Press.
FORD, C.S. and BEACH, FRANK (1951) *Patterns of Sexual Behaviour* New York, Harper & Row.
FORDE, D. and RADCLIFFE-BROWN, A.R. (eds) *African Systems of Kinship and Marriage* Oxford University Press.

FORTES, M. and EVANS-PRITCHARD, E.E. (1940) *African Political Systems* Oxford, Oxford University Press.
FOX, R. (1967) *Kinship and Marriage* Harmondsworth, Penguin.
FREEDMAN, MAURICE (1957) *Chinese Family and Marriage in Singapore* London, HMSO.
FREEMAN, GILLIAN (1969) *The Undergrowth of Literature* St Albans, Panther.
FREUD, SIGMUND (1900) *The Interpretation of Dreams* in J. STRACHEY (ed) *The Complete Psychological Works of Sigmund Freud*, standard edn, vols IV, V, London, Hogarth Press.
FREUD, SIGMUND (1908) *Character and anal eroticism* in J. STRACHEY (ed) *The Complete Psychological Works of Sigmund Freud*, standard edn, vol XIX, London, Hogarth Press (1957-64).
FREUD, SIGMUND (1912) 'The psychology of love' *Collected Papers* vol. IV, London, Hogarth Press (1950).
FREUD, SIGMUND (1923) *The Infantile Genital Organisation: an Interpretation into the Theory of Sexuality* in J. STRACHEY (ed) *The Complete Psychological Works of Sigmund Freud*, standard edn, vol. XIX, London, Hogarth Press (1957-64).
FREUD, SIGMUND (1930) *Civilization and its Discontents* in J. STRACHEY (ed.) *The Complete Psychological Works of Sigmund Freud*, standard edn, vol. XXI, London, Hogarth Press (1961).
FREUD, SIGMUND (1933) *New Introductory Lectures on Psychoanalysis* in J. STRACHEY (ed.) *The Complete Psychological Works of Sigmund Freud* standard edn, vol. XXII, London, Hogarth Press (1957-64).
FRIEDMAN, DR DENNIS (1976) '45 is a dangerous age' *Daily Express* 28 October.

GAGNON, JOHN (1977) *Human Sexualities* Glenview, Ill., Scott, Foresman.
GILLAN, PATRICIA and GILLAN, RICHARD (1976) *Sex Therapy Today* London, Open Books.
GLOVER, LELAND E. (1963) *The Impotent Male* Derby, Connecticut, Monarch Books.
GOODE, ERICH (1974) 'Sex and marijuana' in L. GROSS (ed.) *Sexual Behaviour: Current Issues*, pp. 155-67, Flushing, New York, Spectrum.
GRAVES, R. (1966) *The Greek Myths* Harmondsworth, Penguin.
GREENWALD, H. and GREENWALD, R. (1974) *The Sex Life Letters* London, Granada.
GREER, GERMAINE (1972) *The Female Eunuch* St. Albans, Paladin.
GROSS, L. (ed.) (1975) *Sexual Issues in Marriage* Flushing New York, Spectrum.
GWYNN-JONES, H. (1976) 'The Psychology of Sex' in Hugo Milne and Shirley Hardy (eds) *Psycho-Sexual Problems* Bradford University Press.

HADFIELD, J. (1954) *Dreams and Nightmares* Harmondsworth, Pelican.
HASLAM, M.T. (1978) 'Depression and anxiety in relation to psychosexual disorder' *British Journal of Sexual Medicine* vols 5ff.
HAWESWORTH (1773) *Voyages* vol II, London.
HEEMING, DR JAMES (1977) 'Look-out' *Sunday Times* 8 May.
HIRSCH, E. (1957) *Modern Sex Life* New York, Signet.
HITE, SHERE (1977) *The Hite Report* London, Talmy-Franklin.
HODSON, PHILIP (1977) 'Raising the dead' *Penthouse* vol. 12 no. 5.

ILLMAN, JOHN (1976) 'Sex: are we expecting too much?' *Sunday Times* December.
INGLIS, RUTH (1974) 'Impotence: an examination of man's oldest neurosis' *Daily Express* 4 November.

JOHNSON, J. (1968) *Disorders of Sexual Potency in the Male*, London, Pergamon.
JOHNSON, VIRGINIA and MASTERS, WILLIAM (1975) 'Why working at sex won't work' *Reader's Digest* July.
JOHNSON, WARREN and FRETZ, BRUCE (1974) 'What is sexual "normality"?' in L. GROSS (ed.) *Sexual Behaviour: Current Issues* Flushing New York, Spectrum.
JONES, E. (1918) *Papers in Psycho-Analysis* London, Bailliere, Tyndall & Cox.

KAPLAN, HELEN SINGER (1974) *The New Sex Therapy* London, Bailliere Tyndall.
KATCHADOURIANN, H.A. and LUNDE, E.T. (1972) *Fundamentals of Human Sexuality* New York, Holt, Rinehart & Winston.
KINSEY, AFRED et al. (1948) *Sexual Behaviour in the Human Male* Philadelphia, W.B. Saunders.
KINSEY, ALFRED et al. (1953) *Sexual Behaviour in the Human Female* Philadelphia, W.B. Saunders.
KIRK, G. (1976) Myth London, Cambridge University Press.
KOEDT, ANNA (1970) *The Myth of Vaginal Orgasm*, KNOW.
KOLANSKY, H. and MOORE, W. (1971) 'Effects of marijuana on adolescent and young adults' *Journal of the American Medical Association* April.
KOVEL, JOEL (1978) *A Complete Guide to Therapy* Harmondsworth, Penguin.

LANG, OLGA (1946) *Chinese Family and Society* New Haven, Connecticut, Yale University Press.
LEIDLOFF, JEAN (1977) *The Continuum Concept* London, Futura.
LEMERE, F. and SMITH, J. (1973) 'Alcohol-induced sexual impotence' *American Journal of Psychiatry* vol. 130, no. 2, pp. 212-13.
LEO, JOHN (1977) 'Everybody goes to camp' *Time* 4 July.

LIEBERMAN, B. (ed.) (1971) *Human Sexual Behaviour* New York, John Wiley.
LICHT, HANS (1932) *Sexual Life in Ancient Greece* London, Routledge.
LINACRE, ANTHEA and BOWSKILL, DEREK (1976) *The Male Menopause* London, Frederick Muller.
'Look-out' (1977) *Sunday Times* 8 May.
LYDON, SUSAN (1968) *Understanding Orgasm* Ramparts.

MACE, D. and MACE, V. (1960) *Marriage: East and West* London, MacGibbon & Kee.
MACKAY, DOUGAL (1976) 'Modification of sexual behaviour' in S. CROWN (ed.) *Psychosexual Problems* New York, Academic Press.
MAIN, T. (1976) 'Impotence' in H. MILNE and SHIRLEY HARDY (eds) *Psycho Sexual Problems* Bradford University Press.
MALINOWSKI, B. (1927) *Sex and Repression in Savage Society* London, Routledge and Kegan Paul.
MALINOWSKI, B. (1953) *Argonauts of the Western Pacific* New York, Dutton.
MARRYAT, MARY (1976a) *Woman's Weekly* 29 May.
MARRYAT, MARY (1976b) *Woman's Weekly* 19 June.
MARRYAT, MARY (1977a) *Woman's Weekly* 16 September.
MARRYAT, MARY (1977b) *Woman's Weekly* 24 September.
MARWICK, B. (1940) *The Swazi* Cambridge University Press.
MASSAM, ALAN (1972) 'Impotency — curse of the British male' *London Evening Standard* 17 October.
MASTERS, WILLIAM and JOHNSON, VIRGINIA (1966) *Human Sexual Response* Edinburgh, J. and A. Churchill.
MASTERS, W. and JOHNSON, V. (1967) 'Counselling with sexually incompatible marriage partners' in R. BRECHER and E. BRECHER (eds) *An Analysis of the Human Sexual Response* London, André Deutsch.
MASTERS, W. and JOHNSON, V. (1970) *Human Sexual Inadequacy* Boston, Little, Brown.
MCCARTHY, BARRY (1977) 'Strategies and techniques for the reduction of sexual anxiety' *Journal of Sex and Marital Therapy* vol. 3 no. 4.
MEAD, G.H. (1934) *The Mind, Self and Society* University of Chicago Press.
MEAD, MARGARET (1954) *Growing up in New Guinea* Harmondsworth, Pelican.
MEYER, JOHANN (1953) *Sexual Life in Ancient India* New York, Barnes and Noble.
MILNE, H. and HARDY, SHIRLEY (eds) (1976) *Psycho Sexual Problems* Bradford University Press.
MITCHELL, JULIET (1973) 'Female sexuality: the second Marie Stopes Memorial Lecture' *Journal of Bio-social Science* vol. 5, pp. 123-36.
MORRIS, DONALD (1968) *The Washing of the Spears* London, Sphere.
MORROW, LANCE (1977) 'The great kissing epidemic' *Time* 7 February.

MUDD, J. (1974) 'Physical examination in marital and sexual disturbances' in D.W. ABSE et al. (eds) *Marital and Sexual Counselling in Medical Practice* New York, Harper & Row.
MURDOCK, G. (1949) *Social Structure* London, Macmillan.

NEWMAN, G. and NICHOLS, C. (1960) 'Sexual activities and attitudes in older persons' *Journal of the American Medical Association* vol. 173, pp. 33-5.
NICHOLS, JACK (1975) *Men's Liberation* Harmondsworth, Penguin.
NICHOLS, L.A. (1961) Journal of College of General Practitioners 4.72.

OLDS, J. (1956) 'Pleasure centres in the brain' *Scientific American* vol. 193, pp. 105-16.
OLIVER, P. (1955) *A Solomon Island Society* Cambridge, Mass., Harvard University Press.

PARR, DENIS (1975) 'The state of sexology today' in S. JACOBSON (ed.) *Sexual Problems* London, Elek.
PETERSON, ROBERT (1974) 'Commentary of "Sex and marijuana" ' in L. GROSS (ed.) *Sexual Behaviour: Current Issues* p. 164, Flushing New York, Spectrum.
PFEIFFER, E. et al. (1969) 'The natural history of sexual behaviour in a biologically advantaged group of aged individuals' *Journal of Gerontology* vol. 24 pp. 193-8.
PFEIFFER, ERIC (1975) 'Sex and Aging' in L. GROSS (ed.) *Sexual Issues in Marriage* Flushing New York, Spectrum.
PITT, BRICE (1976) 'Sexual behaviour in the elderly' in S. CROWN (ed.) *Psychosexual Problems* New York, Academic Press.
PLUMMER, K. (1975) *Sexual Stigma* London, Routledge & Kegan Paul.
POPPER, SIR KARL (1968) *The Logic of Scientific Discovery* London, Hutchinson.

RAINS, P. (1971) *Becoming an Unwed Mother: a Sociological Account* Chicago, Aldine.
RORVIK, DAVID and DEVLIN, DAVID (1975) *Women's Medical Guide* London, Book Club Associates.
RUBIN, ISADORE (1965) *Sexual Life after Sixty* New York, Basic Books.
RUDNER, R. (1966) *The Philosophy of Social Science* Englewood Cliffs, NJ, Prentice-Hall.
RYAN, BRYCE (1958) *Sinhalese Village* University of Miami Press.
RYECROFT, CHARLES (ed.) (1966) *Psychoanalysis Observed* London, Constable.
RYLEY-SCOTT, G. (1970) *Phallic Worship* St Albans, Panther.

SALZMAN, L. (1968) 'Sexuality in psychoanalytic theory' in J. MARMOR (ed.) *Modern Psychoanalysis* New York, Basic Books.

SCHOFIELD, M. (1965) *Sexual Behaviour of Young People* London, Longmans.
SHEEHY, GAIL (1976) *Passages* London, Bantam.
SIEGFRIED, ANDRE (1965) *Routes of Contagion* New York, Harcourt Brace & Jovanovich.
SILVERBERG, GERALD (1978) 'Confessions of an impotent man' *Cosmopolitan* May.
SIMONS, G.L. (1970) *A History of Sex* London, New English Library.
STEFANISZYN, B. (1964) *Social and Ritual Life of the Ambo of Northern Rhodesia* Oxford University Press.
STRUBE, GILLIAN (1975) 'A general practitioner's advice' in S. JACOBSON (ed.) *Sexual Problems* London, Elek.

TAYLOR, FRANCIS (ed.) (1978) *Psycho-Sexual Problems* London, British Association for Counselling.
TRIBE, DAVID (1975) *The Rise of the Mediocracy* London, Allen & Unwin.

VAN GULIK, R.H. (1970) *Sexual Life in Ancient China* Brill.
VON KRAFFT-EBING, R. (1899) *Psychopathia Sexualis* London, Putnam (1969).
VATSYAYANA *Kama Sutra,* trans. Richard Burton, New York, Dutton (1962).

WALKER, KENNETH and FLETCHER, PETER (1955) *Sex and Society* Harmondsworth, Penguin.
WALKER, KENNETH and FLETCHER, PETER (1953) 'Non-sexual factors in impotence' *The Medical World* June.
WARE, JAMES (1966) *Alchemy, Medicine, Religion in the China of 320 A.D.* Cambridge, Mass., MIT Press.
WATTS, G.T. (1976) 'Sexual problems following major abdominal surgery' in S. CROWN (ed.) *Psychosexual Problems* pp. 423-31, New York, Academic Press.
WEBER, MAX (1964) *Theory of Social and Economic Action* New York, Free Press.
WOLPE, J. (1958) *Psychotherapy by Reciprocal Inhibition* Stanford University Press.

YULE, DR ROBERT (1978) *Sunday Times* 19 March.

Index

This is primarily a subject index, and does not take account of the numerous references to authors and sources which are to be found in the main text and the notes.

alcohol, 45, 48, 81ff, 89ff, 96, 104, 129
Ambo (Rhodesia), 53
androgen (male hormone), 44
Aristophanes, 58
Aristotle, 134
arthritis, 43
Athens (ancient), 35, 58

biological functionalism, 5-6
Bryant, A, 53

Canton, 55
cardio-vascular (heart) disease, 44
Cauthery, P. and Cole, M, 15
China, 54-5, 59-61
Clement (of Alexandria), 58
cliterodectomy, 3
Cole, M., 76, 78, 149, 155, 162ff.
Columbus, 55
conception control, 24, 34, 79, 87
Cook, Captain, 33

diabetes, 15, 44
de Chardin, Teilhard, 177
Dioscorides, 57

ejaculation, *see* orgasm
Enki, 56

erection/erectile, 9-10, 13, 14, 19ff., 41ff., 44, 45, 47, 50, 57, 59, 77ff., 146-7, 149-51, 154, 176
Esalen, 109
estrogen (female hormone), 44
eunuchs, 61

Family Planning Association, 66, 71, 141
fantasy (sexual), 106, 147-9, 150, 153-4
Finkle, A., 90
Ford, C. and Beach, F., 33
forum, 37, 65, 75, 77
Freud, Sigmund /Freudianism, 18-19, 20, 93, 113ff., 118-19, 123, 129-30, 134, 136-7, 140, 148, 164
frigidity, 11ff., 18, 133

Gillan, Patricia, 76
gonorrhoea, 43, 55
Greece (ancient), 35, 134

Havelock-Ellis, 1
hepatitis, 44
hernia, 43
Hindus, 55
 Indian Vedas, 57, 60

195

INDEX

homosexuality, 6, 28, 30, 34-5, 92, 128-30, 140, 163-4
Horace, 58

illegitimacy, 34
impotence
    definitions, 9ff.
    incidence, in primitive societies, 52ff., in complex pre-industrial societies, 55ff., in modern society, 65ff.
    theories of, 6, 101ff., 159ff.
    treatment/therapies, 160ff.
    see also erection/erectile, orgasm, potency, sex, sex and age, drugs, illness, etc.
incest, 115, 127, 161
India, 59-62
Institute of Sex Education and Research, *see* Cole, M.
Islam, 59
Italy, 70

Japan, 54
Java, 134

Karma Sutra, 1
Kinsey, Alfred, 10, 18, 19, 20, 29, 30, 40, 42
Krafft-Ebing, 1

libido *see* sex drive
Lovedu (Transvaal), 35
LSD, 48ff.

magazines (experience), 2
    see also sex aids/erotica, forum
Mahler, Gustave, 118
Malinowski, B., 52
marijuana, 48ff., 104
Marriage Guidance Council, 52, 66, 69, 141
Masters and Johnson, 12, 15, 18, 41, 81, 122, 127ff., 137ff., 142ff., 152ff., 172
masturbation, 9, 29, 42, 80, 84, 92, 95, 97, 102, 115, 133, 146-7, 148-9, 150
Melanesia, 53
Mesopotamia (Babylonia), 56-7
migraine, 47
Mohave Indians (Arizona), 35
Muhammed, 59
multiple sclerosis, 44
Murdock, G., 33
myotonia (genital), 11, 20
myths
    Mesopotamia, 56
    Hindu, 60
    Egyptian, 56

Nefzawi, Shaykh, 59
Newman and Nichols, 41

obesity, 43, 105, 113
orgasm
    male, 9-10, 13, 16ff., 23ff., 29ff., 38-9, 41, 47-8, 70-1, 133, 143, 146, 150-1, 155, 163
    female, 11ff., 16ff., 23ff., 38, 70, 133
Ovid, 58

paedophilia, 131-2
paraphilia, 35ff., 140
Petronius, 58-9
Pfeiffer *et al.*, 40-1
Plateau Tonga, 53
Pliny, 57
polygamy, 33-4, 60
Polynesia, 33
Popper, Sir Karl, 102
potency, 3, 13, 16, 23, 39, 40, 56ff., 66ff., 104, 116, 134, 177, *see also* erection/erectile
pressure rings, 147
prostitutes (male), 30, 79, 82, 128, 177
prostitution

Indian temple, 3
Phoenician, 3
psychoanalysis, *see*
    Freud /freudianism

refractory period, *see* orgasm

Samaritans, 70
sex and age, 40ff., 73ff., 78ff., 104ff.
sex and drugs, 44ff., 79-80, 81ff., 86ff., 96, 99, 104ff., 129, 154-5, 164-5
sex and illness, 42ff., 104ff.
sex and religion, 56ff., 70, 91ff., 117, 128, 130-1, 164
sex drive (libido), 44ff., 97ff., 104ff., 172ff.
sex roles, *see also* impotence, theories of, 159ff.
sex therapy, 5, 52, 100-01, 127ff., 164ff.
sex aids/erotica, 36, 61-2, 65, 72, 95, 147-8, 174ff.
sex ideologies, 5
sexual intercourse, 9-10, 17, 20, 39, 40, 43, 49, 52ff., 68, 79ff.
sexual surrogates, 77, 149ff., 155

Shaka (Zulu), 21-2
Solomon Islands, 53
Sparta (ancient), 35, 130
Sri Lanka (Ceylon), 54
suicide, 164
Swazi, 53
syphilis, 43, 55, 79

Taoists, 60
testosterone (male hormone), 44, 104
thrush, 43, 96, 107
Thebes (ancient), 35, 130
Theodorus Priscianus, 59
Theophrastus, 57
tobacco, 45, 104

vasocongestion (genital), 11, 20, 23
vibrators, 11, 133, 147
virginity, 34, 54-5
virility, *see* potency
virility contests (Sudanese), 3

Women's Liberation, 6, 18, 63, 69, 172

Zulu, 21-2, 53-4, 56